GETTING IN

A Practical Guide to
Pharmacy School Admission

Throughout the book we give examples of the experiences of students preparing to apply to pharmacy schools, for the sake of illustration and education. Details of these cases, including names, have been changed to protect the privacy of individuals.

While we have done our best to provide accurate information at the time of the book's writing in late 2009, requirements for pharmacy schools are often evolving. Readers are advised to use the worksheets in the book to make sure they have accurate, up-to-date information about the requirements at their schools of choice.

GETTING IN

A Practical Guide to Pharmacy School Admission

What you need to know to get where you want to go

Amber Ault, Ph.D. & Kajua Lor, Pharm.D.

Next Generation Books, a division of Close the Gaps Cultural Consulting LLC

Next Generation Books, a division of Close the Gaps Cultural Consulting LLC
www.closethegapsculturalconsulting.com ~ 608-243-9445

ISBN 978-0-9826053-0-1

Contents

*We dedicate this book to our parents, Pheng and My Lee and MaryLou Ault,
for their loving support and serving as an inspiration to
be the best we each can be.*

*We gratefully acknowledge the University of Wisconsin School of Pharmacy
for all we learned there about pharmacy, community, and health care.*

About the Authors

Amber Ault, Ph.D. is a social scientist with keen interests in institutional transformation around issues of access, inclusivity, and social justice. She holds a Ph.D. in sociology, along with specialized clinical, organizational, and crisis management training in social work, and has published in the areas of race and ethnicity, sex and gender, and mental health. After serving as the coordinator of the University of Wisconsin's Undergraduate Research Scholars program, she became the first Director of Diversity at the UW School of Pharmacy. There she used her sociological training to design strategies that increased the numbers of students of color admitted by and successful in the Doctor of Pharmacy Program, and became more deeply interested in providing cultural skills training to future health care providers. She teaches, writes, and delivers institutional/organizational consulting and individual coaching through her firm, Close the Gaps Cultural Consulting LLC, based in Madison, Wisconsin.

Kajua Betsy Lor, Pharm.D. is a 2009 graduate of the University of Wisconsin–Madison School of Pharmacy. During her pharmacy education, Kajua completed internships with HealthPartners in Bloomington, MN as part of the AMCP/FMCP/Pfizer Internship Program, and with Walgreens in Oshkosh, WI, as well as a clinical rotation in Thailand. At present, she serves as a pharmaceutical care resident at the University of Minnesota's Eastside Family Clinic in Minneapolis, where she uses her Spanish and Hmong language skills to provide medication therapy management and anti-coagulation services to an under-served, diverse population. After completing her residency, Kajua will pursue a career as an ambulatory care pharmacist at an international clinic in the Twin Cities. She has presented her research on Hmong traditional medicine to pharmacy audiences at national conferences, and hopes to continue to educate healthcare professionals on Hmong herbal medicine, culture and health beliefs.

Acknowledgements

I would like to express my gratitude to the colleagues, students, friends, and family members who supported my work on this project. It's amazing how many people there are to thank for assistance with such a short book—another lesson that even small things worth doing usually take a village.

Experience is an invaluable teacher. I am deeply indebted to my colleagues at the UW Madison School of Pharmacy during my tenure as its Director of Diversity, to the students with whom I had the joy to work during my time there, and to my colleagues in diversity work across campus. I especially appreciate Dean Jeanette Roberts for her leadership, openness, curiosity, and optimism; the UW Pharm.D. class of 2009 for their passion; Professor Emeritus George Zograffi, for keen observations and words of kindness; and Betty Chewning , Connie Kraus, and Mel de Villiers for their consistency of vision. Across campus, colleagues in diversity work, including Seema Kapani, Rodney Horikawa, Dang Chonwerawong, Mercile Lee, Rosa Garner, Carmen Reamer, Gloria Hawkins, Louise Root-Robbins, Greg Smith, the L&S SAA crew, MDC committee members, SEED staff and students, and others provided gentle mentoring, support, guidance, and friendship as I learned the ropes; I hope this book will prove useful to your students. I'd also like to express my appreciation to the many pharmacists in the state of Wisconsin who taught me about their profession and endorse the vision of more inclusive and accessible health care. I especially value the time I spent with pharmacists on the admissions committees at the SoP, as well as the chance to get to know Rocky LaDien and Charlie Lee, who both gave generously of their time to support the UW diversity mission.

I am indebted to my writerly friends: Monica Macaulay inspired the idea of a small How To book for pharmacy hopefuls while we worked at Ground Zero Coffee Company in Madison; Nora Jacobson looked at an initial draft at the same coffee shop months later, told me to keep going, and has generously offered publishing advice along the way; Pat Rodriguez offered a careful and productive reading of an early draft; and Carla Corroto has been my beloved friend and writing buddy for 20 years now and is a constant source of good advice, inspiration, comfort, and amusement. Stuart Koblentz, with whom I worked on a high school newspaper in the last century, generously talked me through some important production decisions. AB Orlik, of Writing Barefoot, helped me see the structure of the book more clearly. Carol Bracewell, of Flying Pig Productions, executed its graphic design so that you may see it more clearly, too. Aria Walsh-Felz and Devin Walsh-Felz served as excellent collegiate reviewers. Thanks to each of you.

Finally, I'd like to express my gratitude to others in my circle who have supported this project: Betsy McKenna, Alice Richmond, Lynn Callahan Burns, and Melissa Peyton kindly encouraged forward movement. Kathrina Zippel continues gently to push and pull in ways I appreciate. Meghan Walsh, Rebecca Kemble, and their families have given me both personal support beyond measure and the buttressing of a vision of a more inclusive and socially just world. I was fortunate to receive that vision from my mother, MaryLou Ault. When I told her about my idea for a little book that would especially help first-generation students and students of color pursue their dreams of going to pharmacy school, she said, "I think that's a good idea." So here it is.

CHAPTER 1
Why Are Pharmacists So Darned Happy?

An Introduction by Amber Ault, Ph.D.

When I became the Director of Diversity at the University of Wisconsin School of Pharmacy in January of 2005, I'd only ever known a handful of pharmacists. Over the next few years, however, I interacted with literally hundreds of pharmacists, pharmacy students, and people who aspired to go to school to become pharmacists. I feel fortunate to have met many amazing people among these groups and to have learned a great deal from them about the profession of pharmacy. Among the most interesting things I noticed about pharmacists was something very simple, exciting, and inspiring: pharmacists love their work, and they love their profession.

I can honestly say that I have never met a pharmacist who didn't speak enthusiastically about the profession of pharmacy.

While I have known doctors, professors, teachers, social workers, lawyers, and business people who have complained about their jobs, even while they love their work most days, I have never heard a pharmacist growl about pharmacy. I'm sure it happens, but I have yet to hear it. Instead, I have usually heard pharmacists passionately describe their love for their work and for their profession. Having heard people in other walks of life express their frustrations, I've been taken aback by pharmacists' nearly universal enthusiasm for pharmacy.

What explains the extraordinary career happiness of pharmacists?

As a social scientist, I know that several factors are associated with high job satisfaction. These include autonomy or independence in your work, control over your work day, being adequately compensated or paid for your labor, a sense that your work is valued and respected by others, having work that is intellectually interesting, and having the resources to recover from the stresses of a tiring day. Pharmacy, it turns out, has all of these qualities as a profession.

Pharmacists are currently in high demand, so they can often choose their workplace and set the terms of their employment. And if they discover they don't enjoy working in one setting, they know that, as long as they are competent, they can always move to another job they might enjoy more. One of my favorite colleagues, a pharmacist who became an academic advisor to prospective pharmacy students, used to tell undergraduates that a Pharm.D. degree could open 700 different career paths for them. These range from working in the area of public policy on health care, to conducting research and developing new medications, to pharmacy management, to teaching in schools of pharmacy, and, of course, to working as a pharmacist. And pharmacists work in a range of settings: some own their own drug stores, some work in retail settings like CVS, Walgreens, Target, and Walmart, some work in clinics where patients are seen by other healthcare providers with whom the pharmacist can collaborate, and some work on teams in hospitals, specializing in everything from emergency care to cardiology (heart care) to pediatrics (children's care) to oncology (the treatment of cancer). Some work with insurance companies, determining which medicines insurance will cover. In each of these venues, pharmacists make important contributions, using the technical, scientific, and social knowledge of the profession of pharmacy, and enjoy the benefits of a high-prestige occupation.

Pharmacists earn a median salary of $103,000 (Nemko 2009), so they can afford to accomplish many of their personal dreams—whether those dreams are to help raise their families into the middle class, or to travel the world, or to make important contributions to community organizations, or to do all of these things.

Pharmacists possess great technical knowledge that can be used to help people in a wide variety of ways, and they enjoy learning more as new scientific breakthroughs develop—sometimes as a result of research done by people in the profession of pharmacy. Pharmacists who want to make a difference in communities find ways of doing that—like the Wisconsin pharmacist who got his small town grocery stores to stock health food in order to reduce Type 2 diabetes. Whether they are in pharmacy for the income, the science, the patient care, or the opportunity to contribute to humanity, pharmacists can achieve their goals in their profession. I suspect that is probably why they are such happy people.

When I meet with students interested in pharmacy school, they express a wide range of reasons for considering pharmacy as a career. Below are some of the explanations people have given me over time for their desire to attend pharmacy school:

- "My grandfather owned a pharmacy in a small town, and my dad followed in his footsteps. It's the family business, and I am the next generation to take it on."
- "I will be the last generation of my family to live in poverty. I am the first to go to college, and want a career in pharmacy because it will allow my family's underemployment and economic need to end with me."

- "I love chemistry."
- "I come from an immigrant family, and there's an expectation that I will support my parents in their old age. Pharmacy will allow me to do that."
- "I come from an immigrant family that expects women to be family-oriented. Even though going to pharmacy school and holding off on having kids is non-traditional in my culture, a career in pharmacy will allow me to make enough money even part-time that I can support my family and have a career."
- "I want to help patients."
- "I want to improve the health care system."
- "I want to make a lot of money and have career flexibility."
- "I thought about med school, but can't really handle blood. Pharmacy will let me do science and help people, but won't require dealing with bodily fluids."
- "Doctors diagnose, but pharmacists are on the front line of treatment."
- "Pharmacists helped to save my grandmother's life. I want to be part of that."
- "I met a pharmacist and thought what he did was cool. I'm good at math and science, and thought this would be an interesting career that would let me make a difference."
- "I come from a pharmacy family. I already love it."

All of these reasons give people motivation to take on the challenging work of preparing themselves for careers in pharmacy. All of them are important and interesting reasons to think about choosing pharmacy as a career.

Although it's clear that the pharmaceutical (drug development and sales) industry can be fairly criticized for its extraordinary profit motives, it's also the case that every day, on the front lines of health care, pharmacists are working to get medications into the hands of all of the patients who need them. I have been impressed over and over again by the efforts of pharmacists to assist their patients in extraordinary ways. Over the course of time, I have become a great fan of pharmacists—their dedication, knowledge, and commitment has impressed me deeply. And, of course, there's that undeniable enthusiasm.

During my years in the UW School of Pharmacy, I had the pleasure of supporting the pharmacy school preparation and application processes of many, many students. Some were in high school when we connected; others were college students; still others were people who were returning to school after many years in a first career. Because I am a sociologist, I began to pay attention to the patterns I saw among various groups of students, and to the needs and challenges of students in different groups. In addition to discerning differences among applicants at different stages in their academic careers, I began to notice differences between students who came from "pharmacy families" and those who were the first in their families to enter the profession, as well as between first-generation college students and students from university-educated families, students of color and majority students, and students whose first language is English and those who speak English as a second language. Of course, these designations overlap and are somewhat externally imposed, but they became a lens through which I could focus more clearly on any particular student and anticipate the challenges that she or he might face on the way to pharmacy school. For example, the challenges facing a first-generation college student born in the US are often different from those facing a foreign-born student whose parents were university educated. Students from "pharmacy families" have some special advantages but also some liabilities as they prepare for pharmacy school. Bilingual students have strengths very attractive to pharmacy schools, but if English is their second language instead of their first, they, too, may have some unique challenges.

With careful planning, hard work, a clear vision, good advising, good information, and adequate support, many who dream of becoming pharmacists can become very good candidates for pharmacy school. Knowing the special strengths and the special challenges of students from various backgrounds allows advisors, mentors, coaches, parents, and applicants themselves to develop strategies for maximizing their assets and minimizing their liabilities. I decided to write this little guide with the hope of helping more students prepare themselves as successfully as possible for pharmacy school and for navigating the complicated application process that determines which students are admitted to the ranks and which are turned away.

I invited Kajua Lor, Pharm.D., a recent graduate of the UW School of Pharmacy to join me in this project. While I was coaching students on preparing for pharmacy school and sitting on pharmacy school admissions committees, Kajua was making her way toward her Pharm.D degree. Along the way, she helped many other students who hoped to go to pharmacy school get ready to apply. She served as the president of the university's pre-pharmacy student organization and then as a co-president of the pharmacy school's multicultural student organization, which did special outreach to undergraduate pre-pharmacy students. Between us, we have a perspective that includes both an administrator/advisor's point of view and the perspective of a recently graduated pharmacist. While we agree on the advice we offer here, we have unique experiences, so sometimes in the book we'll make clear that an example or story comes from my experience or from Kajua's. At the end of the book, Kajua offers a summary of her own experience thus far as a happy pharmacist.

Pharmacy isn't for everyone, but for those who hear its call, it can offer a great career. Pharmacy needs more people of color, more bilingual people, and more people with a global sensibility to make health care better. Whether you come from a long-standing US-based family or have only been in the US a few years, whether you are a "first generation" student or come from a family of physicians, whether you are a high school student just beginning to imagine your future as a health care provider or a 50-year-old woman coming back to school now that your children are grown, we think this book will offer you something valuable on your journey.

Welcome. Thanks for reading. Now, let's get started.

CHAPTER 2
Is Pharmacy School for You?

Every year, pharmacy schools turn away thousands of applicants. Those who are admitted to professional programs in pharmacy face several truly demanding years of intensive study. Why do so many people work so hard to become successful in the competition for a coveted seat in a pharmacy school cohort or class? While some people emphasize one element over the other, most people who succeed in pursuing the advanced degree you'll need to practice pharmacy emphasize the following advantages of this career path:

- High income potential and great benefits
- Career flexibility and control over work hours and locations
- A constantly evolving knowledge base that keeps things interesting
- Opportunities to improve people's health—whether through direct patient care, research, drug development, community or professional education, or the development of public policies related to health
- A lifelong engagement with science and math
- The opportunity to work with other medical professionals in a wide range of settings
- The prestige of the profession
- The opportunity to "make a difference," whether by improving the quality of life of one's family, a community, or science itself

Given all of these advantages, you can see why pharmacy is appealing to so many people as a potential career path.

As you decide whether pharmacy is the best professional path for you, it is important to become as clear as possible about your own motivations and specific aspirations for your career in pharmacy. As interesting and as exciting as pharmacy can be as a profession, it's important to realize that many other professions allow people to make a good living, use scientific knowledge, and help people. It's important for you to think about alternative careers that meet your criteria for "a good job" even as you explore pharmacy.

Why?

First, because by comparing pharmacy to other career paths, you will become clearer about what attracts you to this profession and thereby become more motivated to move forward toward your goal of becoming a pharmacist, if pharmacy appeals most to you. Second, it's also good for you to have a back-up plan, in case circumstances arise that require you to change course. Knowing about other careers you could pursue with a background in science and an interest in health will allow you the security of knowing that the education you're getting is useful even beyond a pharmacy career. Third, pharmacy school requires a great commitment of time, energy, and financial resources, so it's important to understand what is involved and whether those demands appeal to you. Finally, as a pharmacist, you will be expected to work on interdisciplinary teams of health care professionals. Knowing as much as possible about the kinds of expertise other practitioners develop will help you appreciate the strengths of pharmacists, doctors, nurses, physical therapists, and occupational therapists, as well as how they complement each other.

How to research possible careers in health care

There are many possible resources for you to use in your research on pharmacy and other possible careers. They include:

Informational interviews. An "informational interview" provides an opportunity for you to ask questions of an expert, in this case an expert in a particular health care field. You may know family members, family friends, the parents of school mates, neighbors, or members of your religious organization who work in health care. These folks are usually flattered when a person asks for an hour of their time to hear about their profession. You may not know anybody personally in each of the allied health fields, so feel free to make some phone calls to request informational interviews. Your own doctor or dentist might be willing, as may someone who practices pharmacy at the drug store in your neighborhood. When you meet with your interviewee, take with you the worksheet we've included in the back of the book for comparing health professions and use that as an outline of issues to talk about with your resource person.

Shadowing. "Shadowing" allows you to spend some time with a person in a particular field while she or he is on the job. Unlike an informational interview, shadowing allows you actually to see and perhaps experience the work a person in a particular field does on a given day. Again, you may want to use your existing networks to arrange shadowing experiences in various health care fields, but if you don't know people who work in health care, it is perfectly acceptable for you to call an office or a clinic in the field that interests you and ask if it might be possible to arrange a shadowing experience. Some places will be more open to this than others, so keep trying if your first request is declined. Some practitioners may prohibit shadowing because of patient confidentiality concerns, in which case an informational interview may be the better choice. Your school or college may have formal shadowing opportunities, so make sure to take advantage of these, as well.

Memoirs and health care texts by health care providers. A number of physicians have written memoirs about their experiences in medical school and in various kinds of practice settings. While not every health care profession has a wealth of such memoirs, almost every profession has books about the history of the profession (pharmacy, nursing, physical therapy, etc.). These books can provide you interesting insider perspectives on these professions, and that can be invaluable.

Professional forecasts about occupations. Just as some people become experts in health care, others are experts in career advising, occupational outlooks, and labor market forecasts. If you are in high school, a guidance counselor can point you toward occupational outlook resources; if you are in college or a graduate of a college that has a career counseling service, the counselors there can do the same. You can find the most recent edition of the *Occupational Outlook Handbook* in public and school libraries. Online, the US Bureau of Labor Statistics (BLS) offers a wide range of resources that can help you sort out what you enjoy and are good at, how these translate into possible career paths, and what the forecasts are for these occupations in the coming years. The URL you'll need is www.bls.gov/k12/index.htm

Compare pharmacy to other health care careers

Now that you know where to look for information about health care careers, it's time to start comparing these occupations with one another. In order to help you clarify what attracts you to pharmacy, as well as how pharmacy rates in your aspirations, compared to other possible professions, we have created two worksheets. The first asks you to rate the advantages and disadvantages of several other professions, from your perspective. The second asks you to list the reasons you are attracted to pharmacy as a career. These worksheets can be found in the final section of the book, and ask you to analyze features of a number of professions and rate how important they are to you. These include pay, hours, intellectual stimulation, career flexibility, worker satisfaction, family friendliness, stress level, diversity, and work environment. We hope you will find these worksheets helpful in determining whether pharmacy is, indeed, the profession for you.

If you decide that pharmacy is for you...

If, after you have done some research on the health professions, you decide to move forward with planning for a career in pharmacy, we hope you'll use this book to support your success.

To become a pharmacist in the US, you'll need to go to pharmacy school. Knowing what pharmacy schools want from their applicants and how to prioritize your time and energy to meet their expectations is the way to maximize your chance of being admitted to pharmacy school.

Pharmacy schools offer academic programs that lead to a degree called the Doctor of Pharmacy or "Pharm.D." degree. In earlier generations, pharmacists earned Bachelor of Science (B.S.) degrees in pharmacy. The new educational standard for pharmacists is the Pharm.D., so if becoming a pharmacist is your goal, this is the degree for you. The academic qualifications required by pharmacy schools vary, though it takes a minimum of six years after high school to earn a Pharm.D. In 2010, it is not required by all schools that you have a bachelor's degree to enter pharmacy school, though more and more people do. It is usually required that you have at least two years of undergraduate college course credits in order to be eligible to apply. Some schools offer six-year programs that students can enter directly after high school. If you know you want to go to pharmacy school, or even if you are unsure about pharmacy but want to keep that option open, the time to make a plan that will maximize your chances is right now.

If you are in high school, this is the time to start preparing for pharmacy school.

If you are about to start college, this is the time to start planning for pharmacy school.

If you are in your college years and have just developed an interest in pharmacy, now's the time to make a plan.

If you finished college some time ago and have now had an epiphany that you would like to go back to school to become a pharmacist, now's the time to make a plan.

The point is: wherever you are in your education, the more time you have to plan for pharmacy school, the more time you have to work on the multiple fronts that will prepare you well. Even if you are only a couple of months away from submitting your pharmacy school applications and have just realized this is the career path for you, making a plan will be invaluable to you in the process of organizing your application. Wherever you are, this is the time to start.

CHAPTER 3
What Do Pharmacy Schools Want?

The sooner you know the qualities pharmacy schools want in their applicants, the sooner you can begin to make a plan of action that will help you prepare to become a great pharm school candidate. So, before we go further, your next assignment is to become very knowledgeable about pharmacy schools and their admissions criteria or requirements.

Your goal here is to become an expert on what schools of pharmacy want to see in their applicants.

In early 2010, there are just over 100 schools of pharmacy in the US. To learn about where they are located, visit the website of the American Association of Colleges of Pharmacy (AACP) at www.aacp.org and click on the "Pharmacy School Locater" link that will allow you to find schools on an interactive map. For a list of US pharmacy schools, visit www.rxinsider.com/schools_of_pharmacy.htm.

One easy way to become an expert on what pharmacy schools want to see in their applicants is to visit their websites. On each website, you should be able to find materials for "pre-pharmacy" students. These materials are generally oriented toward college students, but can provide anyone with a very useful view of what will be expected and of the structure of a school's Pharm.D. program.

If you are still in high school, this information gives you a sense of classes you might seek out, even if those classes aren't required for your high school graduation. For example, if you compare the college classes required for admission by five different schools of pharmacy and see that each school lists "calculus" as a required course, it's a safe bet that learning some calculus in high school will serve you well in your preparation for pharmacy school over the coming years. Taking Advanced Placement calculus will serve you even better.

While you're checking out the websites of schools of pharmacy, explore what these schools would like to see in their ideal applicants in addition to the completion of required courses. For example, do the applications require evidence of community service, health care experience, skills in multiple languages, or cross-cultural sensitivity? Make a master list of all of the things pharmacy schools look at in their applicants. See how common these factors are across schools and what's unique to each school. Doing this allows you to see the academic courses you will need, as well as the other skills, experiences, qualities, attributes, and materials you will need to acquire as you prepare to apply to pharmacy school.

You would be wise to start a file in which you document the things you're doing that are relevant to pharmacy school applications. When you apply—both to your colleges of choice and, later, to a school of pharmacy—you will remember all of the things you have done to prepare yourself. Keep track of community activities, school activities, travel, and any awards or recognition you receive.

Plan for success by mapping what pharmacy schools want

Use this chart to determine what is required of applicants at three schools of pharmacy that interest you, then use this information to make a plan for fulfilling their requirements. You'll find a larger copy of this chart in the worksheet section in the back of the book.

School	GPA	PCAT	Letters	Diversity	Leadership	Healthcare	Application Due Date
1)							
2)							
3)							

COURSES REQUIRED

School	Science	Math	Social science	Humanities
1)				
2)				
3)				

CHAPTER 4

Advice is Nice! Why You Need Good Advising Now

As you now know, getting into pharmacy school is not a simple matter of being a great student—though you will need to be an excellent student. Knowing what pharmacy schools want allows you to plan your academic, extra-curricular, and volunteer life in a way that takes your long-term goal into account. Even though you may be a natural wiz at planning, the more resources you can organize to help you put together various elements of a plan, the more "on target" your outcomes will be. In this chapter, we urge you to make advisors and mentors a key part of the team that will help you get into pharmacy school.

Connect with advisors

It is imperative that you connect as soon as possible with good academic advisors. You'll need a strong pre-pharmacy advisor, and may also need advising support in some of the departments in which you will be taking classes. At a large university, you may have an advising relationship with an undergraduate advisor as well as with an advisor in the pharmacy school. Having input from several advisors can work in your favor, especially if they work well together.

Before you get to campus at your college or university, look at its website to determine whether the school has a pre-pharmacy program, advisor, and/or club. Figure out how to get connected to these resources even before you set foot on campus. Send an e-mail message or make a telephone call to the contact number and make an appointment to meet with an advisor, as well as a pharmacy club staff advisor or student leader, as soon as you can.

Especially important is locating someone on your campus who can give you good pre-pharmacy advising. If you are attending a college or university that has a School of Pharmacy, there will probably be someone in that school who specializes in advising pre-pharmacy majors. Contact the School of Pharmacy at your university, tell someone in the advising office that you are a new pre-pharmacy student, and ask how you could get connected with an advisor to help you design your class schedule for your first year of college. **Make sure to ask that you are put on the school's pre-pharmacy mailing list; this will allow you to**

receive updates on open houses, career days, and other events at the school that may be of interest to you, as well as updates on changes in admissions requirements.

If you are attending a school that does not have a School of Pharmacy on site, don't worry; this is the case for most colleges and universities, since there are only a few more than 100 pharmacy schools in the country. At such a school, there will still very likely be an advisor—either a professional advisor or a faculty member—who specializes in working with students who intend to go to pharmacy school. Again, you'll want to identify this person and contact them before you arrange your first semester's schedule, so that they can guide you in course selection. If you are attending a very small school and can't determine who serves as the pre-pharmacy advisor, ask the staff members in admissions and/or the chair of the department of chemistry or the person who advises pre-med students. Any of these people should have a sense of who, on their campus, is most familiar with the requirements for pharmacy school admissions and helping students to meet those requirements.

If for some reason you cannot identify someone on your campus who is a designated pre-pharmacy advisor or who has experience in helping students from your college go to pharmacy school, you can still get good advising. Because you have researched the schools of pharmacy that interest you, you should know which schools are in your top three. Choose one of those schools and contact it, explaining that you are an undergraduate at an institution that doesn't do pre-pharmacy advising, and that you would like to ask for input as you plan your first couple of years of undergraduate coursework. You could also ask an advisor or faculty member at your school to make this contact for you. Although you are not a student at their institution, many pharmacy school advisors are willing to help undergraduates who will be applicants to their programs in a few years. Indeed, they are often excited to connect with interesting future applicants. **Again, make sure to ask that you are put on the school's pre-pharmacy mailing list, if it has one; this will allow you to receive updates on open houses, career days, and other events at the school that may be of interest to you, as well as updates on changes in admissions requirements.**

How do you know that you've found a good advisor? We think good advising is characterized by the following qualities:

- Good advising is informed by long-term goals but focused on short-term steps toward those goals.

- Good advising reflects a knowledge of the standards and requirements for meeting academic goals.

- Good advising recognizes the relationship between an institution's culture and a student's culture, in order to help the student understand the institution and succeed within it.

- Good advising is clear and straightforward.

- Good advising is honest and positive; good advisors tell students directly about any obstacles they see in the way of particular goals, what students need to do to overcome those obstacles; and how to identify alternative goals, if the student decides to change directions.

- Good advising connects students to various resources that can help them succeed.

- Good advising is smart, compassionate, and empowering.

If you meet with an advisor and do not feel that the advising reflects these qualities, keep looking; meet with other advisors or with staff or faculty members that other students identify as being competent and helpful. Good advising can make an incredible difference in your progress toward your goal, so keep looking until you believe you have found the best resources for you. And remember: it takes a village! We encourage you to recruit and "adopt" several advisors along your way to pharmacy school. Each one will have something special to offer you, and, at the same time, when you hear the same message from multiple sources, you will know it's something to which you need to pay attention.

Build a step-by-step plan

By connecting with an advisor and becoming familiar with the classes you'll need to complete with excellent grades, you can map out the key landmarks in your journey to pharmacy school. This gives you a sense of the big picture of the landscape ahead of you. As the old saying goes, however, "a journey of a thousand miles begins with a single step." It is very important that you begin to break down the big map into a series of smaller, manageable steps toward your destination. This will allow you not to feel overwhelmed by all of the things you need to accomplish in the next few years, and help you to concentrate on really excelling at the tasks before you in any given semester.

The rest of this book is designed to help you think about all of the pieces of that map and how to build a solid pharmacy school application, whatever your experience may be. While it can't take the place of a personalized relationship with an advisor, academic coach, or mentor, it should help you get ahead in your journey toward pharmacy school. We will look at strategies for academic success, preparing for the Pharmacy College Admissions Test, how to arrange letters of recommendation, and how to get the experience you'll need to be a great candidate for schools that want you to have leadership experience, great communication skills, cultural competence, and familiarity with health care. Knowing in advance that you'll eventually be asked to document these experiences on an application will help you think right now about how to develop strengths in these areas—and how to record them.

Before we begin to dig more deeply into these elements of the pharmacy school application, however, we recommend that you take the following steps to formulate a general application plan:

- Identify the deadlines for applications at the schools to which you'd like to apply. Put these dates on your calendar, even if they are two years away.

- Mentally set aside time leading up to those application deadlines to devote to creating excellent applications. The time it takes to coordinate letters of recommendation, prepare application essays, study for the PCAT, and go to interviews is very much the equivalent of a part-time job.

- Set up your schedule for the semester in which you will be applying so that you can integrate these activities without sacrificing your academic success. **It is especially crucial that you perform well academically during the semester you apply to pharmacy school.** That semester's grades will be the latest grades an admissions committee sees, and you want them to be outstanding.

If your college career is already well underway, it is more important that you quickly identify the steps you need to take to create a successful application to a professional program in pharmacy. Here are the steps we recommend:

- Use Chapter 2 to research the requirements of at least three schools of pharmacy that interest you. Take an honest look at your current transcript and how it relates to these requirements. Determine whether you have done well enough in previous coursework both to meet the standards of the pharmacy schools that interest you and allow you to do especially well in future coursework. In other words, is your current foundation strong enough to support you in earning As in the courses that remain on your "to-do" list?

- Locate a pre-pharmacy advisor—whether this is a high school counselor, an academic advisor, or a pharmacy school staff member. Share your ambition to go to pharmacy school with her or him. Ask this person to review your transcript and support you in laying out the steps you need to take to prepare for pharmacy. Discuss specifically whether there are any classes on your transcript to date that you should repeat before moving into additional pre-pharmacy coursework. If your advisor does not know the answer to this question, make sure to contact someone in a school of pharmacy to ask an insider's opinion. Remember that most schools of pharmacy want to see a grade of "B or better" in all pre-requisite coursework. If you earned a C in calculus, it is probably wise to repeat that course and earn an A in it before moving on to calculus-based physics.

- Use this book to create an academic plan with your advisor for the remainder of your academic pre-pharmacy career that includes the pre-requisite pharmacy courses and emphasizes balance over the long haul.

- Use Chapter 6 to develop a success orientation toward the PCAT. Identify when you will take the PCAT or other standardized tests required of applicants to pharmacy school. Create a plan for studying for the exam. Expect to take this exam twice, if you can financially afford to do so; schedule your PCAT so that if you are dissatisfied with your first scores, you may take the test a second time on schedule for your second set of scores to be considered by the admissions committees.

- Use Chapters 8–13 to familiarize yourself with the "non-academic elements" of some pharmacy school applications, including community service, leadership, cultural sensitivity, experience in health care settings, letters of recommendation, communication skills, and other strengths or talents. Begin to think now about how you would demonstrate your experience or ability in these areas. Don't panic! Most people have more experience along these lines than they initially believe. Choose one or two areas that you would especially like to strengthen and begin to devise a plan for doing that.

If you already have earned a college degree and have now decided that you'd like to go to pharmacy school, the steps you need to take are similar to those we've outlined above, although you have some additional considerations:

- Like a current college student, you'll need to identify several schools that interest you and analyze their admissions requirements and deadlines.

- In addition, you'll need to determine whether you completed the prerequisite classes during your undergraduate years, and whether your grades in those courses were strong enough to help you submit a competitive application. If you are missing some classes, or if you didn't give your strongest performance in some prerequisite courses you took, you'll need to address these issues.

- If you are working full time, you will need to determine how many classes you can reasonably take in a semester, given that your goal needs to be performing at an "A" level in those courses.

- Many pharmacy schools will allow you to apply before you have completed all of the prerequisite classes—as long as you can demonstrate that you can finish them successfully before your first semester of pharmacy school begins. If you are a returning student with classes still to be completed at the time of application, you'll need to demonstrate to the admissions committee that you have a workable plan for successfully finishing the remaining classes before you start pharmacy school.

Whether you are a high school student, a college undergraduate, a college grad, or somewhere else along the spectrum, now is the time to build your support network of knowledgeable advisors and to make a plan to get yourself through the front doors of a pharmacy school of your choice!

CHAPTER 5
Achieve Academic Excellence

Pharmacy schools look for well-rounded, interesting applicants who demonstrate strengths in academics and the ability to be compassionate and caring with future patients. It may seem like they want "super-people," and the list of things to focus on may seem overwhelming. The thing to prioritize is academics, because this is the foundation of the knowledge pharmacists must have. If you struggle with math and science, don't be discouraged. Instead, know that these are difficult areas of study that demand a lot of time and attention. To understand them requires work and perseverance. Once you have a strong foundation in these areas, expand your efforts to include other areas that come more easily to you. If your volunteer time, leadership time, sports time, or club time interferes with your ability to perform at an A or B level in math and science, restructure things so that you can devote more time to mastering these subjects. This will pay off enormously as you take the next steps of applying to college, undertaking the college-level classes you need for pharmacy school, and submitting your pharmacy school application. While developing the additional strengths required of applicants is very important, do not allow that task to overshadow your efforts to do well academically. A long list of extra-curricular activities and an average GPA will be far less compelling to an admissions committee than a 3.8 GPA and a focused set of extra-curricular or work experiences.

Now that we've addressed planning for pharmacy school admission in a general way, we'd like to devote one chapter to the most important element in your pharmacy school preparation process, which is academic success. Afterward, in the following chapters, we will turn specifically to addressing the other elements that likely will be part of your pharmacy school application. We'll suggest some useful approaches to these application elements, with the hope that these suggestions will strengthen your strategies and simplify your life at the same time. But first, let's talk about academics.

In earlier sections, we've stressed the role of strong academic preparation and performance in creating a successful application to pharmacy school. We've noted that it's ideal to create a consistently strong record of academic performance, while also pointing out that all is not lost if you have had some difficult semesters, as long as you are able to recover from those. In this section, we share some strategies for developing an excellent academic record. These will work whether you have already created a strong academic history in college, are just beginning your college career, are returning after some time away from campus, or have had some academic difficulties and are now in a recovery phase.

Pace yourself in a way that promotes success

As we suggested in previous sections, pacing yourself so that you can excel is critical, both in your preparation for pharmacy school and during your time as a Pharm.D. student. Many students are so eager to get to pharmacy school that they attempt to take all of the prerequisite courses in math and science as quickly as possible early in their college careers. While we appreciate their ambition, drive, and motivation, too often this approach backfires. Many students who have chosen this route find themselves struggling with academic overload; they may pass the classes they are taking, but they under-perform. So, while they are able to check the required courses off of their to-do lists, their grade point averages (GPA's) suffer. In the end, this becomes self-defeating behavior. Nearly every student applying to pharmacy school will have completed the prerequisite courses, so just finishing the classes will not set you apart from other applicants—doing well in your classes and establishing a strong GPA will.

So, how do you establish a good pace? With the help of a professional advisor, plan your semesters so that your classes have a nice balance: include in each semester some classes that you expect to be in your "academic comfort zone" and some that are more challenging. Try to include in each semester a class that you are taking just for the joy of it. If you are just starting college or returning after a long absence, try to create a schedule that is considered a "light load" at your university. Eventually, you will need to carry at least 14 credits or the equivalent each semester—this is something that pharmacy schools look at because you'll be expected to carry a heavy load in pharmacy school. For starters, however, create a balanced schedule that will allow you to establish a great GPA at the beginning of your career.

Academic pacing: high school

Once you know what pharmacy schools are expecting, try to begin to acquire those skills and experiences as part of your high school education. For example, since calculus likely shows up as a required course for every school of pharmacy, try to take a calculus course in high school. If your high school offers two, take them both. If your high school doesn't offer a calculus course, approach one of your teachers, explain your goals, and ask if he or she could help you figure out a strategy for studying calculus on your own or taking a calculus course as a special student at a local college before you graduate from high school. Many students benefit from taking Advanced Placement (AP) classes in high school, not only because of their academic rigor, but because this allows them to move more quickly through the pre-pharmacy requirements during their first years in college; AP classes allow them to earn college credits before they enter college.

Look at the other elements of pharmacy school applications that you discovered and think about how you might begin to work toward developing these as well. Do you have a chance to study languages in high school ? If so, this is a great way to build language skills and learn about other cultures. Maybe you could join a club that is organized around your language group, take a trip to a community where this is the dominant language, or volunteer for an organization serving speakers of this language. This can give you a great foundation for acquiring skills and experiences that will distinguish you from other applicants to pharmacy school in the future.

If you are already bilingual or multilingual, think about using your language skills in a medical setting or community organization that will let you volunteer as a translator. This kind of experience will help you to demonstrate skills in two areas required by some schools, "cultural competence" and "experience in a medical setting." It will also mean you can speak from experience when it comes time to write your pharmacy school application.

Academic pacing: college

A few universities allow freshmen to enroll on a six-year track to the Pharm.D. right out of high school. If you're seeking admission to such a program, make sure you are well-prepared now.

In their enthusiasm for checking off classes on their academic "to do" lists, many pre-pharmacy students make a crucial error. They take on too much, too soon, without building a solid foundation. As a result, they may finish the prerequisite courses quickly, but their performance in those courses ranges from average to poor. Unfortunately, this then compromises their chances of getting into pharmacy school and/or requires that they spend additional semesters repeating courses or working to raise their GPA's. In addition, whizzing through may set them up for failure in later courses in those subject areas, which just compounds the problem. This, obviously, is a mistake to avoid.

The first way to avoid this mistake is to make sure you are getting really excellent advising—and that you take the guidance of your advisor. Most colleges and universities offer placement tests in some key areas, including math, chemistry, and languages. Sometimes pre-pharmacy students are disappointed—and maybe even angry—when their placement tests put them at a level "below" what they had expected. An unskillful response to this is to deny the test results and an advisor's advice, and to enroll in the course you think you "should be" in. A more skillful response is to look at the placement test results as a gift. If it turns out that your skill in the subject exceeds the demands of the class—that is, the class is easy for you—there's no reason you should earn anything but an A in the course. It will be a nice review for you and allow you to spend a little extra time settling in during the beginning of your college experience. If it turns out that the placement test is accurate, you will be just where you need to be. You'll build a strong foundation

Learn By Example: A STORY

Amalia was a first-year student who was very driven to earn her way as a transfer student into Harvard from the state university in which she was enrolled; her ultimate ambition was to become a cardio-thoracic surgeon, as both of her parents were.

She was enrolled for a light course load her first semester in college, and came to her advisor asking for help in enrolling for two additional courses—demanding courses and additions that created a class load that would have required special "overload" permission. Her advisor suggested she re-think this plan, to keep the three courses she already had, and to earn A's in them, establishing a great academic record that would allow her to make the case at Harvard and build a strong med school application. The advisor declined to give permission to add the extra classes.

The student was very unhappy , and found another university advisor who agreed to grant her permission to carry the 21 credits she requested.

Unfortunately, the semester did not go as well as Amalia expected; she earned B's in a couple of classes and C's in the rest. While these grades are respectable, especially given her course load, they effectively destroyed her possibilities of transferring to Harvard, and created an unnecessary challenge to her goal of going to medical school.

This student had the intelligence and talent to succeed in college and go on into medicine; what she didn't have at that point in her life was the skill of pacing herself, the patience to build a solid academic record, and the wisdom to trust her advisor. She underestimated how challenging the classes she'd enrolled in would be, and she over-estimated her own preparation.

She had difficulty taking the advice of several advisors, and allowed her ambition to drive her to find someone who would support her poor decision to take an overloaded class schedule during her first semester in a new academic environment.

for the next courses and avoid the nightmare of being in a math or chemistry or Spanish class a couple of levels beyond your current competence.

Landing in a class beyond your skill level can lead to poor performance. It can undermine your confidence and cast doubt on whether your dream of pharmacy school is achievable. It is far better for a first-year student to be placed in classes that are a bit "below" his or her current skill levels at the beginning (don't worry—these classes will still challenge you at the end) so that she or he can review, strengthen the fundamentals, and enjoy early successes rather than jump with both feet into courses where she or he will soon be drowning. There will be plenty of time for that later!

A little side note: there is a common belief that if a student hasn't had a lot of advanced math in high school, he or she is beginning college with a deficit, especially when it comes to preparing for pharmacy, with its heavy requirements of advanced math skills. It's also the case that high schools vary widely in how rigorously they teach math and science, so an A in calculus from one school might be equivalent to a D in calculus at another. One of Amber's excellent advising colleagues once told her about two students who were interested in pharmacy school who placed into a developmental math course during orientation testing because their high school preparation was very weak. Although these two young people were disappointed, and may have at first wanted to jump into the standard pre-pharmacy curriculum despite their placement scores, the advisor encouraged them to start in developmental math. The two became friends and study partners, and within three years had completed all of the math pre-requisites for pharmacy school with grades of B or better. The lesson: have the wisdom to start where you are and to build a solid foundation for a profession that will require you to use your math and science skills for a lifetime—and listen to good advisors. **Quality of performance is much more important than how quickly you get things done when it comes to building your academic transcript for pharmacy school.**

Address any bumps in your history: "the turn-around"

Those who provide academic advising to pre-pharmacy students often walk a fine line between dispensing false hope to students with blemished records and giving unnecessary discouragement to students who have had some academic or personal challenges. It is absolutely necessary for you to establish a firm academic foundation upon which you can build your training in pharmacy school; it is also the case that if you have had a difficult semester or two, this does not necessarily mean you have no access to a Pharm.D. education. In this section, we want to talk a bit about how to handle challenges in your past if you see your future being in pharmacy.

First, know that many students have overcome considerable academic odds to successfully achieve pharmacy admission. In her role on the admissions committee at the University of Wisconsin School of Pharmacy, Amber reviewed one applicant who had been dismissed from the university ten years previously for allowing grades to drop to a low 1.2 GPA; a decade later, the student returned and earned a 4.0 GPA in demanding science classes across a couple of semesters, convincing the admissions committee that he was now ready for pharmacy training. She recalls another successful applicant—now a successful pharmacist—who had earned D's and F's during nearly every semester of her first years at a community college. She knows more than one pharmacy student who overcame serious and debilitating illnesses that had affected their GPA's as undergraduates and who have gone on to succeed with their pharmacy applications and educations.

On the other hand, she watched some students who struggled academically resubmit pharmacy applications repeatedly, only to be turned away.

What makes the difference between these two groups—those who struggled but were admitted to pharmacy school and those who struggled but "struck out" in the application process?

The most important difference between these two groups is what we might call "the turn-around." In the case of the student who had been dismissed for poor academic performance, a decade away from the university, an opportunity to work in a discipline-driven institution, and the experience of starting a family gave that student a sense of direction and some very good work habits. When this person determined to go to pharmacy school, he came back to the university and took the undergraduate courses that were required—some of which he failed before, some of which were new to him. He earned A's in every course. While his overall GPA was still very low—about 2.2—his GPA for two difficult semesters of math and science coursework was a stunning 4.0. The admissions committee could see "the turn-around" in this applicant's transcript. What the committee observed was supported by an application essay explaining the change. It was also supported by his references, which described him in extremely positive terms. This applicant had transformed a dismal history into an impressive success.

Similarly, the applicant from a community college who had failed a number of classes in her early college years demonstrated "the turn-around." Her transcript showed several semesters with lackluster grades and then, suddenly, straight A's.

The transcript also showed that the applicant took every science class available to her at her small community college—even classes not required of pharmacy students. What had happened? The applicant's essay described a personal tragedy that inspired her to take stock of her life and set out on a new direction; once she had made that commitment, her grades reflected her ability and hard work. She accomplished her impressive turn-around while working full-time, volunteering, and managing family responsibilities, and her letters of recommendation confirmed that she was bright, diligent, dependable, and a hard worker, just as her transcript demonstrated. Like the previous applicant, she had found the focus and the discipline to use her natural academic talents, and the committee could see that she was resilient and able to handle many challenges, both academic and personal. She graduated from pharmacy school after a very successful student career, and is now in practice in the job she envisioned.

What distinguishes these folks from the people who tried to turn things around but did not succeed?

We think there are two factors. The first, and most important, is focus. Like "the turn-around" applicants, there are many who decide that they would like to go to pharmacy school, assess their transcripts, realize that their grades are weak in required courses, and determine that they will raise these grades. They repeat the courses, but raise the grades only minimally—say from a C to a B-. Sometimes this happens because they are overloaded academically; sometimes it happens because they are working many hours to put themselves through school and don't have much energy left over to study. Sometimes it happens because they are involved with extracurricular activities or have family demands they can't ignore. The end result, however, is that they do not create "the turn-around" in the eyes of the committee. They do not establish that they have laid a new, recent, strong foundation for succeeding in the rigorous coursework required of pharmacy students. Unlike the "turn-around students," they do not demonstrate a dramatic change from under-performing to undeniable success.

The second factor that distinguishes people who have some weakness in their applications but succeed from those who don't is how well they convey to the committee the source of their problems and how they have been corrected. For example, a student suffering from depression during her sophomore year may have had a dip in her grades, and may recover both her health and her GPA by the time she graduates as a senior. If she explains this in the application, the committee has a medical context for interpreting the temporary drop in her performance; if she both explains and demonstrates (with good grades) that she has gotten effective treatment, the committee is likely to see her experience as one that might make her an even better health care provider. If a student consistently has a problem with some area of the PCAT exam—let's say the verbal section—but explains to the committee that English is not his or her first language, the committee has a way of making sense of how a person with a 3.6 GPA and great scores on the math and chemistry sections of the test might under-perform on the language section. If the applicant explains his or her language skills well, and demonstrates fluency in his or her writing and interviews, the committee will likely interpret this student as having something special to offer patients—skills in English and another language—and because the grades and letters of recommendation are excellent, will be less concerned about PCAT scores.

So, to sum up: if you have some sort of deficit in your performance or your profile, correct what you can and explain the situation to the people reading your application. If you decide that you want to go to pharmacy school and recognize that you have some weaknesses that you'd like to correct, correct them full-out. If you earned a C in calculus and decide to re-take it, set your life up so that you can earn an A the second time around—or wait until you can do so. Because you have a bit of a deficit, you need to impress the committee by making a dramatic turnaround. You owe this to yourself, since pharmacy is your goal, and you owe it to your future patients, since we need pharmacists to be expert and confident in the math and sciences that are at the core of modern pharmacy practice.

Become a master planner and study skills wiz

One of the best things you can do for your academic success is to develop good time-management skills and the ability to do long-range planning. At the beginning of each semester, sit down with an academic calendar that allows you to see at least one month at a time (being able to see all of the months of the semester at once is ideal). Look at the syllabus you have for each class and, one by one, put the important due dates and exam dates from each syllabus on your calendar. Put any other important activities coming up in the semester on the calendar, too. Now, look at the semester as a whole and see how things line up. Do you have three exams in one week? Do you have a paper due on the Monday morning after the weekend your sister gets married? Having a sense of how exams, papers, assignments, and additional activities overlap with one another tells you at the beginning of the term how you'll need to work ahead on some assignments in order to be able to succeed at all of them.

Once you have created an overview of the semester's major events, go back to your calendar and schedule in specific obligations. Put all of your classes on the calendar for each week, along with your work schedule, as best you know it. **Now, schedule study time or lab time for each of your classes. You should devote at least two hours of study outside of class for every hour you spend in class. If you are in a history of medicine class that meets for three hours each week, you should put six hours of study time on your calendar for history of medicine—plus time to write papers and finish homework assignments.** Schedule your study time so that it is balanced with breaks and other activities across the course of the week, then **treat your study blocks as though they were appointments with someone important—because they are!** Working in this way will allow you to stay on top of your materials.

Even if the first few weeks of a class seem easy, don't give in to the temptation to skip the study blocks for that class. Keeping these appointments with yourself builds a rhythm, discipline, and the practice of reviewing. Many students make the mistake of thinking that "reading" material for a class is the same as studying it. Studying involves reading the material, taking notes on it, then reviewing the notes, then testing yourself or your study buddies. This is the heart of mastering material so that you will retain it over a long time. Retaining knowledge is important because you will need what you are learning now in pharmacy school; its curriculum builds on the basics you need to master now.

If you would like to learn more about studying efficiently, think about taking a course on study strategies at your university or seeking out one of the many workshops colleges and universities offer on study skills and test-taking. One study strategy that we like is called SQ3R—the Survey, Question, Read, Recite, & Review approach. We have used it ourselves in our own studies and have found that it saves a lot of time and helps to consolidate learning very efficiently. You can read about this approach on-line in several places, including at: www.studygs.net/texred2.htm.

Connect with peers

Because seats in pharmacy schools are limited, you may be tempted to regard other prospective pharmacy students as your competition. While it may be true that your applications will be in the pool at the same time, we'd like to discourage you from adopting an attitude that regards other pre-pharmacy students as your academic enemies. To the contrary, one of the best things you can do for yourself in your pre-pharmacy years is to build strong collaborative relationships with others in your pre-pharmacy curriculum classes. If you do enter pharmacy school with these folks, you will already have a network of colleagues whose strengths you know and whom you can trust in difficult times. The people who fare best in pharmacy school—and in life—are people who work well with others, so now is the time to start building your network.

How do you do that? Invite people in your classes to study with you as you work your way through the pre-pharmacy curriculum. Be generous with what you know: often, we have seen that the students who teach others during study sessions often excel on exams; rather than being a waste of their own time to help others, they have the advantage of reinforcing the material for themselves as they clarify it for friends. In this way, generosity pays off—not just in cementing friendships, but in raising your own level of comfort with material.

Don't be afraid to reveal your own weaknesses in group study situations. Over a long stretch, each person will need help and will give it. One of us learned the hard way, when she was struggling with statistics, that it was a grave mistake to assume she would be of no value to a study group. As a result, she holed up for the semester and failed the course, while other students working in groups passed. If you struggle mightily with a subject, you are providing other people an opportunity to learn to explain the topic clearly. And: you will be able to repay their kindness in another course when you have strengths that they need. By sharing these struggles with others, you will build a solid community of friends upon whom you can call throughout your undergraduate and professional school years, and likely throughout your life, as well.

Connect with professors and teaching assistants

Getting to know your professors and teaching assistants (if you are at a large institution) can be immeasurably helpful to you during your pre-pharmacy years, as well as in pharmacy school. Many students don't realize that many faculty members and teaching assistants enjoy meeting with students outside of the classroom. As a result, students don't make an opportunity to get to know them or only visit them after trouble develops in a course. These students, unfortunately, often find themselves at a disadvantage when it comes to creating a competitive pharmacy school application. Those students who get to know their faculty members enjoy the following advantages: additional support, encouragement, and practice in mastering the material of a course—which, of course, helps create a successful GPA; the opportunity to receive coaching and mentoring from someone with more years of success in academia; the chance to build community on campus; and the creation of a long-term relationship in which a faculty member gets to know you in a way that will allow her or him eventually to write a detailed, sophisticated letter of reference for you when you apply to pharmacy school.

Our suggestion is this: toward the beginning of each semester, make an appointment to meet with each of your faculty members. When you meet with your professors, let them know why you're interested in their classes, what your background preparation is, and that you are working hard to succeed. Ask if they have any recommendations for studying successfully—perhaps even asking what their own experiences are with regard to study strategies. Ask if you might come back from time to time to discuss the content of the class and questions you may have. Of course, it is important that you do this sincerely—if you are not sincerely interested in the course, this will be apparent to the faculty member and will not work in your favor. Do check in with the faculty member whenever you are having difficulty mastering the course's material or having trouble working it out on your own or with your study group. Always approach faculty members with an attitude of respect and curiosity.

Even if you encounter a setback in a class, it is important to view this as an opportunity to learn new skills. A few years ago, Amber taught a small class for pre-pharmacy and pre-med students who were college freshmen. When the class received their first papers back, many students had earned grades below what they expected and below what they were accustomed to receiving. One young man had been the valedictorian of his high school, and had never before received a C on an assignment. He was, of course, both dismayed and upset. Still, he handled the situation with maturity and a productive approach. He wrote to Amber and asked for an appointment, saying, "the grade I earned was lower than I expected, and I'd like to learn how to improve my writing so that I can do better on future assignments." During their meeting, the student was cheerful and focused on developing an understanding of what he could do differently. He ultimately earned an A in the course. Just as importantly, he impressed Amber with his maturity, dedication, and interest in learning. When he asked for a letter of recommendation a few years later, as he was planning to go to Medical School, she was happy to write a reference that was glowing and full of these kinds of details. This is how to make lemonade from a little bit of lemon juice!

Locate first-year resources

Many universities and colleges offer special learning opportunities to first-year students. These programs range from "learning communities" to undergraduate research programs to mentoring programs that will allow you to connect with other students and faculty members who have experience in your areas of interest. These opportunities can be important for a number of reasons:

- They give you a chance to build relationships that will allow you to feel more at home at your college or university.

- Those relationships can help promote your academic success by creating a network of study buddies and mentors who can give you insider information about how to succeed in demanding pharmacy coursework.

- Research opportunities can give you an applied understanding of the theoretical concepts you're covering in your classes, and this can make the learning easier.

- Many pharmacy schools appreciate applicants with experience in research and community-oriented campus programs.

- Making these connections early allows you to build a base for letters of recommendation from people who can say they know you well by the time you apply to pharmacy school, whether that is in your sophomore year in college or after you graduate.

Find additional support

Like the student who approached his professor after he got a C on a paper, the best students are often those who use college and university resources to their full advantage. Explore whether your school has a writing center, a chemistry support center, a program for first-generation college students, a general tutoring service, a math club, or other opportunities to get additional support and training. We are always amazed at the students who bypass these resources, because these resources often help B students become A students and A students achieve excellence beyond their teachers' expectations; those same students eventually often go on to serve as tutors themselves, which allows them to consolidate their own learning, feel good about helping others, and further develop their leadership resumes. It's often C or D students who insist on toughing things out on their own, thinking that there is a stigma attached to getting tutoring or assistance. Trust us: all of the best students do it!

CHAPTER 6
PCAT? What's That?

The Pharmacy College Admission Test (PCAT) is a standardized, timed examination that every pharmacy school will require you to take. This test helps admissions committees compare you with other applicants on your academic abilities. If you have already taken the ACT, SAT, or other standardized, multiple-choice oriented examinations, you will have some sense of the design of the PCAT, which is divided into several sections focused on different areas of knowledge. The PCAT is a test of your knowledge—not your potential, or aptitude—so the more course work and other kinds of preparation you have before taking it, the better you are likely to perform. In addition, the PCAT is a measure of how well you do on these kinds of tests, so the more you practice the skills involved, the stronger your scores are likely to be.

It's important for you to do your best on this exam; although some schools evaluate applicants holistically and see the PCAT as just one factor, many still focus on two main variables in evaluating your application: 1) grades in your pre-pharmacy courses and 2) PCAT scores. As we have indicated elsewhere in this book, it's possible to get into pharmacy school without strong PCAT's—but the truth is that it is much harder to do so. We want to encourage you to do what you can to maximize the possibility that you will do very well on this exam. This is especially the case if there are some rough spots in your academic record or if you come from an institution that is not regarded by others as especially academically rigorous. Scoring well on the PCAT under those circumstances will put to rest any questions about whether you are capable of performing well in pharmacy school.

Some people simply enjoy multiple choice exams more than others. Some people have more experience with them. If your undergraduate institution is a liberal arts college, you may have been through a demanding science program that never asked you to take a multiple choice test. Your last standardized exam may have been the ACT in high school. If you know you are inexperienced with multiple choice tests, have test anxiety when facing these sorts of exams, or anticipate language or cultural barriers that might slow you down on the test, it's even more important that you begin as early as possible to prepare for the PCAT. In this chapter, we offer some strategies for doing just that.

First, of course, get acquainted with the exam. Go to www.pcatweb.info for the most recent PCAT updates and free information about the exam. Write down the exam test dates and print the "Candidate Information Handbook" to learn about exam locations, what to bring to the exam, the registration process, and what happens after you take the exam. The PCAT is offered multiple times per year. We suggest taking the PCAT early. If you are dissatisfied with your score the first time, you will have a better idea about the exam and have a chance of doing better next time. From your research on your schools of interest, you will know whether they have a minimum required PCAT score, what the average PCAT score among students in their recent incoming classes has been, and whether the PCAT is one of many factors the application reviewers examine or one of only two—that is, how much weight a particular school gives your performance on this exam.

At the time of this writing, there are a total of 240 multiple choice questions on the PCAT and two essay sections. Each multiple choice/multiple guess question has four possible answers; only one of the answers is correct. Your job is to identify the right answers to each item. If these kinds of exams make you nervous, remember these two truths: 1) the answer is right in front of you, already on the paper; and 2) you have a 25% chance of randomly guessing the right answer. The more familiar you are with the material, the more practice you have with these kinds of questions, and the more calm you are when you take the exam, the better your chance of identifying the right answers. The test is divided into separate sections which have different time limits. You will have four hours to complete the test.

The PCAT score is calculated from the number of correct answers, so make sure you don't leave anything blank. It is better to guess on an item than to skip it; leaving an item blank results in no credit; a guess gives you a 25% chance of a right answer. If you can eliminate two of the four possible answers, your chances are even higher. Your score will list the scaled score and the percentile rank for each of the multiple choice subtests and all the total multiple choice tests combined. You will be assigned a composite scaled score and percentile scores for the overall exam. Percentile scores indicate the percentage of students who scored below you when you took the test. If you have a composite percentile of 62 it means that you scored higher on the PCAT than 61% of a "norm group." There are also two scores for the writing section; these are reported as raw scores on a scale of 1 to 5. Five is the highest score possible.

Prepare to do your best on the PCAT

So, what can you do in advance of the exam to make sure you give it your all?

- Do your best in all of your classes. The PCAT is designed to test you on the content of courses in the pre-pharmacy curriculum common to many schools. The more you really absorb and retain from your classes, the more you remember for the PCAT.

- Identify your weaknesses and improve them. If you know you are weak in English, for example, get help. You could do that by taking additional classes, hiring a tutor, getting self-study books on grammar, or signing up to work with someone at the writing center on your campus. If you are a new speaker of English, consider finding a "conversation partner" who will help you master the language more quickly. If you know you are weak on multiple choice tests, get more practice and address any test anxiety issues.

- Purchase (or borrow from the library) a PCAT study guide. And use it! Copy or scan any practice tests and answer sheets before you take them so that you can use them again. Plan to take practice tests several times before your first PCAT.

- Take on-line PCAT practice tests that you can find by "googling" them.

- Remember when you are taking on-line or pencil-paper practice tests that it is really important to time yourself just as you'll be timed at the exam. The more often you practice this, the better your sense of how long you can spend on any question will be. In addition, you will become better and better at recognizing patterns of questions on the exams.

- Ask the pre-pharmacy advisor at your college if she or he helps students prepare for the PCAT.

- Consider starting a PCAT prep group.

- Explore private PCAT exam preparation courses. It is not necessary to take one of these to do well on the PCAT, and they can be expensive. Nonetheless, we have known many students whose scores improved significantly with the help of these resources.

- Ask around to see if you might know someone who has materials from a private PCAT prep service that they could share.

- Find and use preparation materials for the "Millers Analogies Test." This will help to prepare you for some of the complicated verbal reasoning items on the test.

Suggestions for taking the PCAT

- Get enough sleep the night before the exam. Cramming definitely will not help.

- Wear comfortable clothes.

- Be prepared. Know where the testing site is. Bring the correct identification and supplies, including your No. 2 pencils.

- Make sure you have enough time. Keeping a good pace will help so that you don't rush.

- Finish all the questions you do know and go back to the questions that were hard for you.

- Don't change answers unless you are absolutely sure that the answer you chose first was incorrect.

- Make sure you completely erase incorrect answers on the answer sheet.

- Plan to leave cell phones and all other or electronic devices outside the testing room.

- Don't leave answers blank! The score you get is based on all the questions you got right.

- Try to stay calm. Know that if you aren't pleased with how you do this time through, you can try this test again in the future.

What to do after the PCAT

After you take the PCAT, you will probably have a sense of how well you did. Unfortunately, this sense may be very accurate or highly inaccurate. You may feel you did poorly but later discover you did quite well. Once you have taken the exam, try to focus on something much more controllable: your progress in any classes that you are taking that semester. Remember that while the PCAT is important, it will not likely make up for mediocre grades in classes you're taking right before your application to pharmacy school. If your grades are outstanding, a committee may be more likely to accept an average PCAT score. The reasoning? Past performance is the best predictor of future performance. So, if you have a very strong academic record and something goes awry with the PCAT, you're in a better position than if you have average grades and a great PCAT performance. Of course, the ideal is to be strong in both.

If, when your PCAT scores arrive, they are similar to the average recent scores of students at the schools to which you are applying, particularly on the math and science subtests, you may decide not to take the test a second time. If your scores are lower than the average at your schools of choice, or below any established minimum, you will likely need to take the test again. Analyze where you did poorly and think about how you can improve. Analyze how you prepared the first time and plan a new strategy for preparing the second time. Return to the practice tests; take them until you feel very comfortable with the exam. This can be hard to do while you are a full-time student or working or parenting, but it is worth the investment of time if you want to see your scores improve. It's important not to despair, but instead to figure out what about your previous strategy for preparing was not effective and to do something different. Many students improve their scores significantly the second time they take the exam.

If you take the exam a second or third time and see no marked improvement in your score, and feel you have used every possible strategy available to you to prepare differently, it is probably time to take a break from taking the exam. Again, it is important to not allow this experience to become demoralizing for you. Focus on the successes that you have had in your academic life and recognize the strengths in your application. Focusing on these will allow you to present your credentials to the admissions committee in a way that focuses on your strengths. If your academic performance is strong, your letters are positive, you have accumulated health care and leadership experience, and your application essays are written carefully and with attention to detail, it is likely that a reviewer, too, will see your excellent potential as a pharmacist.

In order to help reviewers understand your portfolio better, if you have struggled with the PCAT but are strong in other areas, it will likely benefit you to make a comment on your PCAT scores in the application. You can do this in a section of the application that allows additional comments, or in a letter to the committee. If you struggled with the PCAT because English is not your first language, so its analogies still "trip you up," it would be important to convey this to the reviewers. If you come from an excellent liberal arts college where the science classes all demanded papers and essay exams, so you are out of practice with this exam format, that might be worth saying. If you suffer from test anxiety that is most acute under timed situations, it would be helpful for the committee to know this. If your PCAT scores are not as strong as your grades, the more the reviewer can contextualize your PCAT scores in the bigger picture of your life, the more comfortable the reviewer will become with the idea that your grades are a better indicator of your abilities than the PCAT.

To sum up succinctly: one of the best things you can do to prepare for the PCAT is to excel in your pre-pharmacy school courses; the best thing you can do if your PCAT scores are not as strong as you wish is to excel in your pre-pharmacy school courses!

Check out the chart below for a structural summary of the components of the PCAT. To learn more about the specific contents of each section, go to www.pcatweb.info.

The Structure of the PCAT

Sub-Test	Questions	Time
Verbal Ability	48 questions	30 minutes
Biology	48 questions	30 minutes
Chemistry	48 questions	30 minutes
Quantitative Ability	48 questions	30 minutes
Reading Comprehension	48 questions, 6 passages	50 minutes
Writing	2 passages	30 minutes per passage

CHAPTER 7
Break It Down and Build It Up: The Application

Now that we have talked about the profession of pharmacy, planning to make yourself a strong applicant for a pharmacy school, strategies for academic success, and how to get ready for the PCAT, we turn to the application itself. In this brief chapter, we provide a set of recommendations for presenting a great application. In the remaining chapters, we address in depth several of the individual areas of the application that you may encounter.

Your pharmacy school application has many disparate elements: references, essays, transcripts, PCAT scores, and interviews may all be part of the material you are expected to provide. Below, we offer some recommendations for managing your application efficiently and successfully.

Recommendation 1: As far in advance as possible, preview the applications for the pharmacy schools that interest you. Doing this several years in advance is not too soon! Although the application may change between now and when you apply, having an advance sense of what's expected of you will be invaluable. If you are applying to pharmacy schools this year, the sooner you can take a look at the application, the better. If the application is available only on-line, open your application early and print the individual sections, if possible. If this is not possible, contact the admissions director and ask for a paper copy of the application for your use.

Recommendation 2: Determine whether your schools of interest require stand-alone, individualized applications or whether they subscribe to the Pharmacy College Application Service (PharmCAS). PharmCAS serves as a centralized application service for schools of pharmacy and the students applying to them. About 70 percent of pharmacy schools use PharmCas as their standardized application coordinating resource, while the remaining 30 percent request direct applications to their programs (Figg & Chau 2009). You may wish to apply to some schools that use PharmCas and some that request unique applications. Visit the PharmCAS website at www.pharmcas.org to preview the process of submitting materials to PharmCAS and the schools that use this service.

Recommendation 3: Become familiar with all of the deadlines associated with the application: deadlines for your materials, for references, and for PCAT scores are all important. Determine whether the schools that interest you use "rolling" application deadlines and conduct a rolling review of applications or whether they have one firm deadline. For schools that conduct a rolling review, plan to submit your application as early as possible.

Recommendation 4: Become familiar with all of the expenses associated with the application: application fees, transcript fees, admissions fees, etc. If you are in need of scholarship support in paying these fees, contact the admissions director at the school and ask if the application fees can be waived and what you need to do to apply for a scholarship or waiver. Begin to budget now for the application fees and interview travel expenses you'll need to cover several applications.

Recommendation 5: Start thinking now about who you'll ask for references, and alert them early in the process (see the chapter on "References" for more specifics).

Recommendation 6: Study the questions for the application essays in advance. Set aside time to work on these essays leading up to the application deadline. Make sure you give yourself time to draft, re-write, and edit these essays. Try to find an academic tutor, writing center staff member, or classmate with good editorial skills to give your essays a once-over. Make an appointment or two well in advance of the application deadline to have someone give you feedback on your essays. Do not, however, "borrow" any material from another applicant or former applicant; this may risk your career.

Recommendation 7: Make sure you complete all sections of the application, including any section that asks for "additional information." Use the "additional information" section to let the reader know more about why you want to attend pharmacy school, why there's a weak spot on your application that you have now overcome (for example, your PCAT scores are low because you took the test in a second language, but your grades are all fine; your grades dropped your sophomore year because you were caring for an ill relative, but your grades have recovered now, etc.), more about your personal history, or what kind of pharmacy practice you'd like to specialize in.

Recommendation 8: If the application gives you room to elaborate on answers, provide more than lists. For example, if the application asks about your leadership experience, don't simply list "Susan G Koman Breast Cancer Race for the Cure participant" (which is not necessarily "leadership") but explain that you "organized a weekly training group of women living with breast cancer to participate in the Race for the Cure," if this is true, because it lets the reader know how your participation in the race did actually involve leadership.

Recommendation 9: Make sure your application is free of typographical and spelling errors.

Recommendation 10: If an area of the application doesn't work well with your situation—say it asks for five academic references and you have been out of school for 10 years—**contact the Admissions Director about your situation and ask if there are alternatives.**

Recommendation 11: Check out the materials related to pharmacy school admissions and degree programs created by the American Association of Colleges of Pharmacy at www.aacp.org/resources/student/pharmacyforyou/admissions/Pages/PSAR.aspx. The AACP also publishes a text version of its entire report; you may be able to get this at your university library.

Recommendation 12: If you are re-applying to a school after having not been admitted on a previous attempt, make sure that you demonstrate in your application that you have taken the advice the school has given you for improving your application. This shows the committee not only that you are a stronger candidate, but also that you take direction well and respect the committee's guidance, which is something pharmacists value.

CHAPTER 8
Write Your Way Into Pharmacy School

During the course of your pharmacy school application process you will be asked to write a surprising number of essays. These will include polished, formal "personal statements" focused on why pharmacy school interests you, as well as essays on leadership, cultural competence, or issues in the profession of pharmacy. They will also include informal extemporaneous essays you'll be asked to write "on the spot," by hand, during your pharmacy school visit. Avoiding writing is not a good reason to choose pharmacy school!

Still, many students attracted to pharmacy school have had educational experiences centered less on writing than on the skills needed in most math and bench sciences courses. As a result, unless you come to pharmacy as one of our favorite pharmacists did, with an undergraduate degree in speech and theatre, you may find the writing involved with pharmacy school applications a little daunting. In this chapter, we offer some recommendations for writing excellent essays as part of your pharmacy school applications.

Why do schools of pharmacy want you to write essays?

Schools of pharmacy include essays in their application criteria for a number of reasons. First, admissions committees are interested in the broad category of "communication skills" in their applicants, and written communication is part of this. Pharmacists use their writing skills to convey information about patients to other professionals, to present research findings to the practice community, and to communicate with staff members, colleagues, and superiors. In a profession as technically sensitive as pharmacy, clear, concise, accurate ways of conveying information are critically important. In addition to allowing committees to assess applicants' writing skills, however, essays allow reviewers to develop a more personal sense of a student. Knowing what attracts the person to pharmacy, which experiences the student has found challenging, transformative, or valuable, and what he or she hopes to do with a Pharm.D. degree helps a committee assess how a school's program might benefit that individual—and how that individual's presence in a class might benefit the community of the school.

It pays to approach your essays with great care. Many promising applications have been rejected because their author treated the essays casually. In a detail-oriented profession like pharmacy, reviewers pay attention to where you place your commas, whether you write in fragments, and whether you have developed creative new ways of spelling common words (you lose points for that!). On the other hand, essays that are thoughtful, well-written, well-organized, technically flawless, and substantively interesting earn the respect of reviewers.

As with other elements of the application, the sooner you know what you're expected to do, the sooner you can begin to think about how to do it—and to line up the resources to do it well. Here are our recommendations:

- Determine as early as possible how many essays you will need to write for each application, the topics about which you'll be asked to write, and the parameters of each essay. For example, does a school specify how many words are the minimum and maximum for any particular essay?

- Begin to develop your essays as early as you can. Allow enough time to develop several different essays. Make an appointment in advance of the application deadlines to meet with a tutor at a writing center or to have a colleague who has good editing credentials review your early drafts. Ask these readers to point out to you the most interesting aspects of your essay, so that you can develop those ideas or topics further. You may also want to consider hiring an independent writing coach or application consultant to review your materials.

- Make sure your essays are focused, well-organized, and reflect who you are.

- Make sure your essays are technically flawless.

- Work on your essay drafts in a word processing program; avoid procrastinating so long that you feel you must write in the application's on-line essay window and submit a first draft to the committee. The committee will know whether it's seeing a first draft or a third or fifth.

- Avoid overly-flowery or complicated language. Avoid using words you don't use in daily conversation; the reviewers will be more impressed by sincere and straightforward expressions of ideas than by "big words" that don't convey clear meanings.

- A cultural note: if you are not familiar with the standard "five paragraph keyhole" model of essay writing common in the US, learn this form and apply it to your admissions essays. This model includes an introductory paragraph, three paragraphs in which you develop different aspects of your theme, and a concluding paragraph. It works well in many situations, and the formula can be modified to fit smaller assignments, such as paragraph-length essays. For example, reduced to paragraph size, this model would include an introductory sentence, three or four sentences developing the main point, and a sentence or two in conclusion.

- The instructions for your application essay may say "this work should be your own," but that does not mean you cannot receive editorial feedback on your essays. Taking your essays to a tutor or editor will help you successfully express yourself and help you develop stronger writing and editing skills. You are being compared to many other people who have sought out extra help with their writing! Hiring someone to write your essays for you or "borrowing" someone else's essays is, of course, strictly off limits.

- Make sure you are answering the question or fulfilling the assignment. If you write an essay for PharmCAS on "why I want to be a pharmacist," resist the temptation to submit it again in answer to the question "how will you enhance the diversity of the pharmacy program at our school?" on a stand-alone application. This gives reviewers the impressions that a) you did not read the question carefully; b) you are too lazy to write an original essay for each application; and c) you believe the reviewers are not going to read your essay or allow it to affect their rating of your application. These impressions will work against you in the review process, given that there are many applicants who clearly follow the instructions and invest much time and care in their essays.

- Any time an application offers you an opportunity to write, take it. For example, if an application includes a space for you to share "anything else you want us to know about yourself," make sure to use this space. Any commentary you include there should be as polished as the formal essays you submit in the other areas of the application.

CHAPTER 9
How to Round Up Great References

Whether you are currently in high school, college, or the work force, this is the perfect time to begin thinking about your letters of recommendation to pharmacy school. The earlier you begin to prepare for this part of your application, the less stress you will have during the application process.

The first step we recommend is determining how many letters of recommendation your schools of interest require, and from whom they want to see recommendations. Most schools require multiple recommendations and specify that a particular number of these come from your university or college faculty. They may further designate how many should come from professors in the sciences and how many should come from faculty members in other disciplines. In addition, some schools place considerable value on having recommendations from pharmacists or other health care providers familiar with your abilities and/or from people who have supervised you in volunteer or work environments. Knowing in advance what your goal schools require in terms of letters of recommendation will allow you to plan in advance to arrange for the recommendations that will allow your application to be considered complete. It's crucial that you know whether each of your schools wants letters of recommendation to come directly to the school or to go to PharmCAS, and what the associated deadlines and processes are in each case.

Academic references for current or recent students

Ideally, you will have had recent positive experiences in classes with faculty members who will be happy to support you in pursuing your goals. Remember that each of your teachers, lecturers, and professors received help from others who wrote letters of recommendation for them, and they are usually happy to support students in pursuing their dreams of going to graduate or professional school or starting a promising career.

If you are just entering college, we encourage you to stay in touch with your teachers, mentors, coaches, and supervisors from your high school days. You may wish to include one or more of these people among your references, if your goal schools allow it. In addition, as you begin your college career, it will benefit you to be mindful of your ultimate desire to comfortably ask your professors, lecturers, or Teaching Assistants for letters of recommendation. There are a number of ways that you can help your faculty members help you when it comes time to ask them for letters of recommendation. We outline these below:

Strive for academic excellence. Most important, of course, is to work hard and perform well; establishing a strong academic track record will make it easier for your teachers to feel confident that you can successfully handle the academic rigors of pharmacy school.

Get acquainted. Although a strong academic performance may be the basic criterion for a faculty member to use in writing a letter, when a teacher has a sense of who you are as a person, she or he can usually write a letter that will be much more interesting to an application committee. The committee will see many candidates with excellent GPA's, so the more you can become a memorable individual among those, the better. By allowing your teacher to connect your face and your name, see how hard you work and how well you interact with others, and understand a little about your background and life, you allow that person to both feel a sense of connection to you and have details that will allow him or her to write a stronger letter. How do you let your teachers know you in a positive way? Here are some strategies:

- Attend class regularly; arrive on time; sit in the front rows; raise your hand to make intelligent contributions to class that indicate you are prepared and interested.

- Visit the faculty member or TA during office hours. It's okay to make an appointment just to get acquainted early in the semester. This will make it easier to connect with the teacher should you need help in the class or simply want to have deeper conversations about the course than class time allows. Be respectful of the faculty member's time during office visits.

- Again, do great work. Papers that are carefully written, tests that show evidence of hard work and creative thinking, and assignments that reflect thoroughness and care attract the attention of those who read them.

Be kind: Although most pharmacy school applicants are outstanding students, being an excellent student is not the only requirement. Most health care training programs want to see evidence of kindness, compassion, and care in the students they admit, because these are important qualities in health care providers. Amber still remembers the letter of recommendation for an applicant who was a strong performer in biochemistry class, and who had the support of her biochem professor—not just because she was a hardworking, bright student, but also because the student kindly assisted her each day with her coat and books when the professor came to class after breaking her arm. That simple act of human kindness made the student remarkable to her teacher—and to the admissions committee.

Academic references for those who already have college diplomas

While there are many advantages to taking some time away from school between your undergraduate years and starting pharmacy school, one of the disadvantages lies in the difficulty that returning students sometimes face in fulfilling the reference requirements at schools with very specific requests for academic references—for example, for three academic references from science faculty. Folks who have been studying in other fields—for example, we know a number of students who went to law school between undergrad and pharmacy school—may have access to recent faculty references but in areas that aren't science-focused. Applicants who have been in the work force but not in school may have abundant work references, and some of these may even be science-focused, such as those for candidates who spent several years working in the pharmaceutical industry—but are still challenged by the requirement to have letters from faculty. Faculty members may have retired or moved on to other institutions; students may have been taught by TAs who have now graduated or left the university, or applicants may feel that so much time has passed that a faculty member will not remember him or her well enough to write a letter of support. Below, we provide some strategies for addressing these situations.

First, if you find that you need to take a few classes now in order to shore up your academic record as you prepare to apply to pharmacy school, you'll be in a position to ask those faculty members for letters of recommendation. Second, even if you don't need to complete any prerequisite coursework, you may have decided to take an upper-division math or science course to demonstrate to the admissions committee that you have retained or gained competencies in math or science during your time away from the university. If you take this approach, you will have an opportunity to ask the faculty member teaching these additional courses to write a reference on your behalf.

Ask your goal school for clarification and whether there are exceptions for people returning after years of work or study in another field. By contacting the admissions director in your goal school, you accomplish a couple of tasks: first, you find out whether the admissions committee allows returning adult students to substitute some work-related references for some faculty references; second, you let the admissions staff get to know you a little bit—which is why it's important to be polite and thoughtful during these interactions, even if you discover no exceptions or substitutions can be made.

Research whether your former faculty members are still at the college or university where they taught your classes. If so, it becomes easier for you to contact them. If not, all is not lost: if you expect that the person will remember you, chances are that the chair of the department can tell you how to contact the faculty member now. It's also possible you can find him or her using a search engine like Google.

Prepare materials to help your potential reference remember you and see that you did well in his or her class. When you contact a faculty member after an extended period, it will be helpful for that person to see your resume and maybe your pharmacy school personal statement; ideally, they can also review your transcript. If you live near the university where the faculty member works, it should be possible to set up an appointment to deliver these things in person; if you are at a distance, plan to send what you can as e-mail attachments when you first write to this person, and to send the remainder via regular mail.

Contact the faculty member and remind him or her when you took his/ her class and the grade you earned, and let him or her know about your pharmacy school plans. If you can make an appointment to do this in person, do so; otherwise, use phone or e-mail to make your request. Again, deliver or attach relevant documents, and provide the faculty member with information about deadlines, forms, etc. so that the faculty member will be able to assess whether he or she can honor your request.

If you cannot find your faculty member: Sometimes, a faculty member dies or becomes disabled, or leaves the country, or has separated from a department in a way that was difficult for the person and the university. In a situation like this, consider approaching the chair of the department in which the faculty member or graduate student taught. Let the chair know about your hopes to go to pharmacy school, your need for academic references, and your performance in the class of the faculty member who is unavailable. If you can provide a resume and supporting materials, the chair may be willing and able to write a letter on your behalf because your performance in his or her department was excellent, even if she or he didn't directly have you as a student in class.

Non-academic references

Some schools will allow you to submit non-academic references as part of your application. If this is the case, think strategically about who you will ask for a reference. You may wish to ask an employer or former employer, someone who supervised you or worked with you in a volunteer setting, someone who was your coach on a team, an advisor to a student organization in which you were a member, or a leader in a religious community in which you participate. While your academic references should be able to speak, at the very least, about your intellectual skills, your academic strengths, your integrity as a student, and your potential to succeed academically, non-academic references often round out the picture of who you are for an admissions committee. In this section, we think a little more about two separate categories of non-academic references: employment references and non-employment references.

Employment references. Pharmacy admissions committees are very interested in employment references for several reasons. First, pharmacy is a profession, so the ultimate goal of any pharmacy school is to prepare you to join the profession as a competent, skilled, contributing worker. It is possible that on the admissions committee there will be a pharmacist or two, and she or he will read applications with an eye toward whether you sound like someone he or she would like to hire. Second, work references often comment on issues about which academic references are silent—whether a person comes early and stays late (or comes late and leaves early), whether the person works well with others, whether he or she shows initiative and makes contributions to the workplace, etc. Third, admissions committees often read academic performance in light of a person's work obligations. For example, if a student is working 20 hours a week and paying for college herself or himself and her GPA is 3.2 instead of 3.6, the student will be evaluated more favorably than if he or she earned a 3.2 GPA but was not working; this is especially true if there are strong letters from an employer. Finally, if an applicant reports working in a pharmacy or other health care environment, the committee will be very interested in the perspective of a pharmacist or other health care professional about the applicant's potential to succeed in health care. **If you have worked in a health-related setting or in a lab setting, it's important to have a letter from someone there;** to report employment experience in a health care setting but have no letter of recommendation from the supervisor will only raise eyebrows (except if your supervisor is your parent, in which case, you need to explain why you didn't ask for a letter).

Non-employment references. Non-academic/non-employment references may come from people who have supervised you in a volunteer capacity, coached you on a team, or observed you over a long time in some context in the community. If you ask someone to write a non-academic/non-employment reference, make sure that the person you ask knows you well and understands that this recommendation is very important to your future. Let the person know that it is okay to provide the committee with details and examples of their experience with you. Sometimes reference writers are tempted to simply "check the boxes" on reference forms; while this fulfills the requirement, it does you a disservice, because it represents a missed opportunity for the committee to learn more about you.

Mistakes to avoid

- Don't deny that you need to collect references! While you may be working on your application right down to the deadline, you need to give references more preparation time; ask early and don't be afraid to send a reminder close to the deadline.

- Don't choose someone who doesn't know you. The best remedy for this is to make sure your teachers get to know you; the next best is to provide them with details they don't know about you but can use in reference letters via resumes and personal statements.

- Don't choose someone who doesn't write well. If you work in a pharmacy and realize that your assistant manager is more verbally fluid than your manager, or more likely to take some time working on your reference, it may be better to ask the assistant manager for the recommendation, even though he or she has less "status."

- Don't choose someone who may say something inappropriate, like suggesting a relative will make a large donation to the school if a particular applicant is admitted.

- Don't fail to sign the confidentiality form/access waiver. In order for the admissions committee to take your references seriously, they need to know that the people who recommended you felt free to speak freely. Signing the form that says you waive your right to read your letters allows them to have this confidence.

How to ensure great recommendations

- Do become familiar now with the references required by your goal schools.

- Do ask references in advance.

- Do supply your references with everything they need—forms, URL links, resumes, transcripts, personal statements, envelopes, and stamps.

- Do ask directly, "Would you feel comfortable writing a positive reference for me?"

- Do ask for more references than are necessary. If one falls through, you're covered; if the school ends up with one or two more than are necessary, they won't generally count this against you.

- If you have trouble supplying the specific kinds of references required by your goal school, do contact the admissions director and ask for her or his recommendations about alternatives.

- Do sign the confidentiality form that allows your references to write confidentially to your schools of choice.

CHAPTER 10
Do You Have Health Care Experience?

Many schools of pharmacy include "experience in health care" among the elements of the application for admission that they will evaluate. Some schools require health care experience; others simply recommend it. When health care experience is recommended but not required, an institution will accept applications from students who do not have health care experience, and will evaluate the lack of health care experience in the context of your broader application. If you are very young and have only completed a year and a half of college at the time of application, and you have a great GPA and strong PCAT scores, the admissions committee may be forgiving. On the other hand, they may say, "this is a great application, but we have others with similar GPA and PCAT scores who also have health care experience." Ideally, you will have some form of health care experience before you apply to pharmacy school.

Pharmacy schools encourage students to get experience in health care for many reasons. One administrator at a large state university pharmacy school that required it for admission told us, "We want applicants to have experience in health care because we need to know they will be comfortable around people who are sick; it would be unfortunate for someone to invest in four years of pharmacy training and then discover that they can't be around people who are ill." Of course, not all people who earn Pharm.D. degrees end up in direct patient care positions—as we've said earlier, there are many things to do with a pharmacy degree—but this Dean had an important point. Even if you intend to go into public policy or pharmacy management or drug development, you'll likely spend a year of your life in clinical internships as part of your pharmacy training, so it would be good to know that you'd be somewhat comfortable working with patients, even if for a short time.

Fortunately, there are many ways to arrange to have health care experience prior to your application to pharmacy school.

Perhaps the most obvious way to get health care experience, however, is one of the most challenging: getting experience in pharmacy practice. Let's talk about that first, then move on to other venues in which you might be able to gain health care experience.

Because you intend to apply to pharmacy school, gaining experience in a pharmacy practice setting is a great opportunity to develop a sense of familiarity with the profession that appeals to you. Many pharmacies hire "pharmacy technicians," people who work under the direction of pharmacists, filling prescriptions and greeting customers, and checking them out at the cash register. The jobs often pay well and give pharmacy techs an excellent familiarity with the workings of a pharmacy. Unfortunately, because these are excellent jobs that are in high demand, they are also difficult to find. If you can obtain a pharmacy technician's position, this will serve you well in your preparation for pharmacy school, assuming you are able to limit your work hours so that they do not interfere with your academic success. Some students, for example, are able to work as pharmacy technicians during summer and winter breaks or for a few hours each week during the school year. These positions help students grow familiar with medications and patient care, and they help pharmacy technicians get to know pharmacists who can speak or write on their behalf as they apply to pharmacy school or to jobs after graduation.

Sometimes, students can't obtain pharmacy tech jobs as high school students or undergraduate college students, but can work as cashiers or general clerical staff members in a pharmacy. This, too, offers an opportunity to see how pharmacies work and to become acquainted with pharmacists. Some students we have known have worked as clerical staff members in retail stores such as Walgreens, and even if they were not hired to work in the pharmacy, these jobs allowed them to fill in for pharmacy clerks and cashiers in a pinch, which opened the door to pharmacy experience for them.

Fortunately, there are many interesting legitimate venues for acquiring health care experience on your way to pharmacy school. Some of these are obvious, while others may involve a little more creativity on your part. Some obvious opportunities include either working for pay or as a volunteer in any of the following venues:

- Nursing homes
- Hospitals
- Doctor's offices
- Community health clinics
- Community vaccination/health programs

Some of the less obvious opportunities might include:

- Working at summer camps that include kids who have medical issues
- Volunteering for the Special Olympics in a substantive way
- Participating as a peer-educator in a campus health education program
- Volunteering at a homeless shelter or domestic violence shelter or suicide prevention hotline
- Working as a personal assistant to a person with disabilities
- Volunteering with a hospice program
- Providing translation services to family or community members who need assistance during medical appointments
- Participating in summer healthcare education programs for future providers
- Providing care to ailing family members
- Participating as a member of a research team working on an applied health project (one in which you would have some patient contact)
- Arranging shadowing experiences and/or informational interviews with pharmacists in your community (this is not health care experience per se, but shows an effort to become acquainted with the profession)

While it's nice when applicants can be compensated for their experience in health care, having paid employment in a health care setting is generally not necessary in order to demonstrate some health care experience. The important goals are to

- Demonstrate your sincerity about working in health care
- Demonstrate that you have learned something of value to your future career during these experiences
- Acquire some skills, insights, and curiosity that will support your work as a pharmacist

Admissions committees read applications carefully, so do your best to be accurate about your experiences—neither understating them nor inflating them. For example, an applicant who presents participation in a marathon as part of the health care resume because she or he raised funds for the American Cancer Society by running the race is likely to be seen as "reaching for straws." An applicant whose only health care experience begins a month before the application deadline will be seen as playing to the application; this may be overlooked by the committee if the student is very early in their college career, but this may also be a "tie-breaker." Ideally, you will acquire some long-term involvement in a health care setting, even if on an intermittent, volunteer basis (for example, working with special needs swimmers at the YMCA every summer), prior to your application to pharmacy school. You will be able to identify what you have learned from that experience in the essays you will write for your application. **Getting the experience is not enough—reflecting on it thoughtfully is what will distinguish you from other applicants.**

We have created a worksheet for you to use to document and analyze the health care experience you have had so far, and to plan for the kind of experience you'd like to get between now and when you apply to pharmacy school. Find it at the end of the book in the worksheet section.

CHAPTER 11

What Is Cultural Sensitivity and Why Do Pharmacists Need It?

Your pharmacy school application may ask you to demonstrate something called "cultural competence" or "cultural sensitivity" or "cross-cultural experience." In this section, we offer you some strategies for preparing to respond to these sections of applications, no matter your background or experience. Cultural competence is an area in which we all have strengths and in which we all have room to improve.

Why do pharmacy schools care about cultural competence?

Let's talk first about why schools of pharmacy, along with other training programs for health care providers, have begun to express an interest in the cultural skills of their applicants. There are many reasons for this, but the greatest one relates to producing a generation of practitioners that has technical, scientific, and clinical skills but also very strong patient relationship and communication skills. In order to provide excellent patient care, clinicians need to have the personal and cultural skills to work effectively with people from diverse backgrounds—and this means being able to work well with both patient populations and the colleagues, supervisors, and supervisees with whom a clinician will interact. Developing strengths in the area of cultural sensitivity affects both the quality of patient care and the business "bottom line;" as a profession, pharmacy is increasingly aware that working well with diverse populations is not just good pharmacy practice but also good business. Although some schools of pharmacy include cultural competence training in their curricula, the truth is that this is still an evolving part of many schools' training programs. By selecting applicants who are already in the process of developing cross-cultural skills, admissions committees can maximize the chances that the pharmacists they eventually graduate will be people with an awareness of the importance of culture and cultural differences in health care.

Despite the great importance of cultural skills to any clinician, students often find themselves confused when asked to talk about their experience, preparation, and skills in the area of cultural competence or "diversity." This feeling of uncertainty is common for students who come from backgrounds we describe as "monocultural," or ethnically non-diverse, as well as those from backgrounds we describe as "multicultural." If you're feeling nervous about this part of your application, you're not alone. Our goal in this chapter is to ease your anxiety, give you some strategies for assessing your cultural experience and awareness, and help you think about ways of effectively talking about your current level of cultural competence in your pharmacy school application.

For people whose backgrounds are monocultural

Many of us grow up in environments in which we have limited exposure to people different from ourselves. Our community members may all have the same racial and ethnic heritage, the same religious or spiritual practices, one language (such communities are often described as "monolingual"), and predictable ways of going about life. Being raised in such an environment means we are likely to become intensely competent in our culture of origin, learning its finer points from the inside. On the other hand, it can raise our anxiety when we encounter people from other religions, language groups, cultures, sexual identity groups, class backgrounds, etc. Particularly if we have been raised to be more fearful than curious about people different from ourselves, it can be overwhelming to try to figure out how to become more skillful or comfortable with people whose life ways differ from our own.

Fortunately, even if you come from a monocultural environment, you have many resources on which to draw to increase your awareness of differences and how they might affect health care. For example, even if you were raised in an all-white, middle-class, Norwegian-descended community in the Midwest that was home to your parents and your grandparents before them for several generations, you will still have been exposed to some diversity. In your community, for example, there are likely to be elders, middle-aged people, and youth, and each of these groups is likely to experience and see the world differently. You have probably already seen and experienced these differences, observed some conflicts across these groups, and watched how these groups could cooperate with each other. You may have observed people with various sorts of disabilities within the community; some people in your community may have had physical disabilities, while others may have had cognitive disabilities or mental illnesses. These forms of difference also require interpersonal skillfulness on the part of community members if a community is going to be "inclusive." Think about the kinds of diversity that you may have encountered in your community of origin and the strengths that you may have developed there that you can build upon now.

Beyond personal experience at home, many people raised in monocultural environments expand their cultural skillfulness through interactions with people of cultures different from their own when they attend college, work in bigger towns or cities, or travel across the US and in other countries. Many of us develop our first awareness of cultural differences through friendships with people from other cultural backgrounds—whether these are "pen pal" relationships, friendships with college roommates, dating relationships, international host family duties, or joining study groups that include people of a variety of backgrounds. Sometimes these relationships happen intentionally and sometimes they happen through "circumstance," but, either way, becoming personally acquainted with people whose backgrounds and life experiences are different from our own is an important and legitimate way to expand our cultural awareness and sensitivity.

There are also many other ways to incorporate a quest for cultural knowledge into your life. Studying a language other than your "first" language is a great way to get to know about another culture—and being fluent in more than one language is a significant advantage to you as a future health care provider. Traveling in ways that allow you to interact with the people who live in the places you visit (as opposed to going to a resort in another country and only interacting with the resort staff) provides another great opportunity to interact with others whose cultural frame of reference is different from our own, and to begin to see how our own life ways are not necessarily "right" or "better" but simply a reflection of our cultural histories. Visiting museums, cultural festivals, concerts, and workshops can also raise your level of cultural awareness, knowledge, and sensitivity.

Books, films, plays, and other educational media can serve as vehicles for learning about diverse populations within the United States and in other regions of the world. Academic areas of study that often open students' eyes to issues of culture and cultural differences, in addition to the study of languages, include anthropology, sociology, social psychology, African American, Asian, and Hispanic studies, women's studies, literature, and ethnobotany. In addition to offering classes in these areas, most colleges and universities engage in cultural programming to introduce students to issues of interest to various communities and populations. Most also host multicultural student organizations, such as Black Student Unions, Pan-Asian Alliances, and Lesbian, Gay, Bisexual, and Transgender (LGBT) organizations that are frequently welcoming of students who consider themselves "allies" of these populations. You may even be able to participate in a multicultural pre-pharmacy, pre-med, or allied health organization on your campus as a way of educating yourself further about issues of culture and health and building friendships with other students interested in these issues.

So, if you come from a monocultural environment, it will be important for you to consciously seek out education and experiences around issues of diversity in order to help prepare yourself for pharmacy school, and there are many ways of doing that. As you respond to this area of the application, it is okay for you to acknowledge that as a person raised in a largely Asian community you had few opportunities to make friends with white people before college, and that you came to college with stereotypes about whites that have been challenged as you have studied with, roomed, with, and befriended white people, and that you now can see how it is important for you to understand white cultures more deeply because, as a health care provider, you will likely have many white patients. It is less effective to say that you have had a job at a pharmacy that "serves a diverse population" or that there were customers from many backgrounds who came into a store that employed you, because these statements don't give the reader a sense of what you learned from your experiences. **It is not enough to be in the same vicinity as people from other backgrounds; you must be paying attention to what you can learn from them.**

Again, remember to think broadly about diversity. Interesting application essays on cultural competence can center on working with kids with disabilities, elders, and patients living in poverty and extreme wealth, as well as on differences along the lines of race and ethnicity. One of the most interesting essays on cultural competence Amber recalls focused on an applicant's experience working as a pharmacy technician in a pharmacy that had several customers who were in the process of transitioning from one sex to another. The applicant very respectfully described how new and curious this was for her, how she was uncomfortable at first with these patients, and how she needed to learn how to ask simple questions of her patients in order to serve them well. For example, she needed to learn how the person would like to be addressed—as "Mr." or as "Ms." She wrote thoughtfully about the need of patients to feel comfortable with their pharmacists, so that they could ask questions and get good care, and how it was her responsibility as a member of the pharmacy staff to earn their trust. Although this applicant had not had the opportunity to work with many people from racial backgrounds different from her own, the committee could see that she had the basic curiosity, skills, and respect that would allow her to ultimately work well with patients from across a broad range of populations. **Your goal is similar: it is not to become an expert on every culture but to become the kind of curious, thoughtful, respectful**

person who will continue to learn what you need to know about the patient populations you will encounter in order to serve them well over the course of your career.

For people whose backgrounds are multicultural

Applicants who are members of "historically under-represented groups" may have a stronger experiential base for responding to application questions about diversity than applicants from monocultural backgrounds. Nonetheless, applicants who come from racial/ethnic minority groups, who have disabilities, who come from minority religious groups or from countries outside the US, who are bilingual or multilingual, who are first-generation college students, or who are members of the lesbian, gay, bisexual and transgendered community, face special challenges in responding to questions about their cultural skillfulness. In this section, we review some of those challenges and make recommendations about addressing them.

The challenge of stating the obvious. One of the biggest mistakes students from historically under-represented groups make in addressing "cultural competence" questions on pharmacy applications lies in their tendency to overlook obvious features of their life experience that have allowed them to develop cultural competence. Sometimes this reflects a "culture of humility" that has taught the student not to draw attention to himself or herself; sometimes this simply is an oversight—because you are immersed in cross-cultural interactions, it can be hard to see them as significant—you just take them for granted.

For example, some students who are bilingual or multilingual fail to mention this on their applications, or mention it only in passing, by mentioning that they have informally provided medical translation services to members of their community. Most pharmacy school applicants are monolingual, and pharmacy is in great need of bilingual and multilingual pharmacists, so this is a skill that any applicant should emphasize if she or he has it. Sometimes, students from ethnic minority cultures forget to mention that they are intimately familiar with their own cultural group. While you may assume that it should be obvious to an admissions committee, it is important to spell this out for a number of reasons. Again, because pharmacy is in need of practitioners familiar with minority cultures, this is an asset to you as an applicant; it is also the case that some people of minority descent are not raised in minority communities, so unless you make it clear to the committee that you are familiar with a particular minority group (Latinos, South Pacific Islanders, African Americans, Croation refugees, etc.), the committee can only guess whether this is the case, and that usually works to an applicant's disadvantage.

Something else that many applicants from minority cultural groups, the LGBT community, first-generation populations, and the pool of students with disabilities often neglect to mention in their applications is that **because they belong to a minority group, their experience in mainstream institutions almost always constitutes cross-cultural experience.** It is important to remember that "cross cultural" experience is not just the experience of people with majority racial standing interacting with others from minority groups; from the perspective of a minority person, interacting with members of the dominant or majority group requires cross-cultural skills. To be a person of color in a mostly white institution, a first-generation student in a school where most of the other students and faculty come from formally educated families, a student raised working class in a middle-class university, a gay, lesbian, or bisexual student in a mostly straight school, a trangendered or transsexual student in a hetero-normative environment, or a student with disabilities in an institution built on presumptive non-disability means a person must frequently engage in the process of learning a different culture and working with/learning from people very different from yourself. This is a legitimate form of cross cultural skill-building that few minority applicants point out in their diversity essays. If this is your experience, point it out in your application!

While minority students may already have a wealth of cross-cultural experience as a result of their interactions with people from majority groups, it is nonetheless important for you to seek out additional training and experience in this area. While an African American student may have extensive experience with whites, she may have had little or no exposure to Latinos/as, people form various Asian communities, or members of the multiracial lesbian and gay community. An immigrant from Croatia may be very familiar with Croat and Serbian cultures, and may have had interesting cross-cultural experiences with white US citizens, but may not yet have had opportunities to learn about Black history in the US. Identifying areas in which you can strengthen your cultural awareness, knowledge, and skills, and then pursuing experiences and education in these areas, can only help your pharmacy application and your preparation as a pharmacist. It is important to document these experiences and efforts, along with the experiences you have had in your own community and in interactions with the cultural majority, in your application materials.

Prepping cultural competence questions: what everyone should know

In order to help you prepare for the cultural competence areas of the pharmacy school application, we are including two documents at the end of this book. The first is a list of ways to increase your cultural competence; the second is a cultural competence self-assessment to help you think more clearly and specifically about your current areas of cultural awareness, your awareness of issues of diversity and inequality, and the areas in which you may want to seek out more education and skills related to cultural competence.

CHAPTER 12
Show Off Your Leadership Experience

Your pharmacy school applications may ask you to demonstrate your leadership experience, skills, and qualities. In this chapter we talk about why leadership skills are important for pharmacists, various ways you might think about leadership in the context of your application, and how to communicate your leadership skills. We also offer a worksheet at the end of the chapter to help you clarify your leadership experience and goals you may have for acquiring leadership skills.

Why are pharmacy schools interested in leadership qualities among applicants?

At first glance, it may seem surprising that pharmacy schools require applicants to demonstrate leadership skills as part of their application portfolios. After all, success in pharmacy school primarily depends upon the ability to succeed in challenging academic courses based in math and science. Many people may have a stereotype of a pharmacist as quiet and bookish, and not necessarily as a highly social person or a leader in his or her community. As you learn more about the profession of pharmacy, however, you will come to understand the importance of leadership within the profession, as well as the leadership role that pharmacists play in health care and in their communities.

There are several ways in which pharmacists exercise leadership skills. First, as recognized experts in a specialized area of patient care, pharmacists are expected constantly to develop expertise in their field and share this expertise with their patients and colleagues—an important form of leadership. Second, pharmacists often work on interdisciplinary teams composed of physicians, nurses, and social workers, and need to be able to contribute to those teams in competent, skillful ways—another important form of leadership. Pharmacists also serve as advocates and advisors to the health care industry and to governments, providing leadership in the areas of health care policy. Within the profession of pharmacy, pharmacists participate in a range of professional organizations and many serve in leadership roles within those organizations, which advance care, monitor standards within the profession, and provide ongoing training to pharmacists. Finally, pharmacists often use their leadership skills within communities—whether by doing outreach at community health clinics, educating youth about the profession of pharmacy, or designing projects that support their community's health and well being.

During the time Amber served as the Director of Diversity in a pharmacy school, she took a camping trip to a rural northern part of the state. On a trip into town, she stopped at the grocery store and was surprised and impressed to discover a very large, well-stocked health food section in what looked like a big-box grocery in a very small, rural town. After shopping, she went across the street to a local café and struck up a conversation with the owner. When the owner learned where she worked, the owner started to tell her about the great pharmacist the town had. Amazingly, the owner asked if she had seen the health food section at the grocery. The owner told her that the pharmacist in town had become very concerned about the rates of Type 2 Diabetes in the area and had begun to do educational outreach designed to reverse and prevent it. He realized that in order to support patients in living healthier lifestyles, they would need to have access to the healthier food he was advocating that they eat. He went to the local grocery and convinced them to develop a healthy-eating section by assuring them he would be sending patients in to purchase these products. As a result of his efforts, the town was moving in a healthier direction. Clearly, this is a profound kind of leadership—one that puts patient and community health above any profit the pharmacy might have seen from selling more insulin.

Formal and informal leadership

The first thing you think of when you're asked to describe your leadership experiences, qualities, and skills may be the formal offices, titles, or roles you hold or have held in organizations. These are important, but they are not the only way to demonstrate leadership. Indeed, many students underestimate their leadership skills on pharmacy applications because they have not held "official" titles. I have often seen this to be true especially of first-generation students, women students, and students of color. In this section, we talk about both formal and informal leadership experiences that may be of interest to a pharmacy school admissions committee.

If you are at the point of filling out your pharmacy school application, you will want to list under the leadership section any formal leadership roles you have held previous to the date of your application. If your application deadline is still some time away, you may want to think about taking on a formal or official leadership position in an organization before you apply to pharmacy school. While admissions committees will likely be impressed if you have served as an officer in an organization, they will also want to know something about what you accomplished in that role. They will sense fairly quickly whether your "office" was "on paper only" or whether you made significant contributions during your time as a leader in an organization. If you are reflecting on past experiences, be sure you can articulate your contributions; if you are about to take on new leadership roles, make sure that you have the time and energy to make a real difference in the arena in which you are providing leadership.

Official roles in volunteer organizations or teams. You may demonstrate formal leadership on your pharmacy school application in a number of ways. It will be a feather in your cap if you have served as the president of a pre-pharmacy student association, but only so many students can have that role; admissions committees recognize this, and also realize that leadership skills are very transferable. If you have been the captain of a sports team or the captain of your "Neighborhood Block Watch," or your Residence Hall Council, or the Employee Resource Committee at your workplace, the committee will know that others have recognized your leadership skills at school, in the neighborhood, or at work.

Leadership in your workplace. You may never have had a formal office in student government, your church, or a community organization. Many students working their way through school juggle school, work, and family in lives that don't leave much room for student or community organizations. Nonetheless, you may have demonstrated leadership in a work environment that will impress an admissions committee. If you have been a student worker, perhaps you have been promoted to a tutor trainer or lead TA or lifeguard coordinator in your work on campus. If you work off-campus, perhaps your colleagues have elected you to head a committee or your supervisor has asked you to train new employees in skills in which you are accomplished. Maybe you have organized an annual company outing or party—a task that takes good organizational, communication, and team-building skills. Think not just about your official title and role, but about instances in which you have worked to improve situations in your workplace, guided other workers, and initiated new events, processes, or programs. All of these build your leadership skills and demonstrate them to a committee.

Leadership in your community. Your community at this point in your life may be the community of students in your classes, program, or campus, the neighborhood in which you live, a faith community, an ethnic or sexual identity community, or all of these. You may have engaged in leadership in these domains without having been elected to a formal office. Indeed, true leadership often expresses itself in the actions of people who simply see a need and work to address it. Amber remembers one pharmacy school candidate who had organized a study network for international students at her undergraduate institution. She was an immigrant and an outstanding student herself, and wanted to help others learn how to succeed in a US academic context. She helped many students, and organized tutors to help many more, though her work was never set up as a formal student organization. When she first applied to pharmacy school, she didn't mention this incredible effort. There were two reasons for this oversight: first, she came from a "non-bragging" culture, and it didn't seem appropriate to her to draw attention to this effort; and second, because she had no formal title or role, it didn't seem "official" enough to her to mention. During her second application to pharmacy school, she outlined this work in detail, and was subsequently admitted. A review committee can only know about your leadership experiences if you tell them! Again, it is important to think not just about official titles, but about the skills and actions that exemplify true leadership.

Leadership in your family. Just as many students discount the informal leadership roles they play in their communities or schools, many may neglect to mention the leadership roles they play in their families. If your family is a first-generation family in the United States, particularly if your family came from a country where the dominant language is not English, you may have spent considerable time and energy helping your family adjust to the US. You may have served as an informal translator at medical appointments and school conferences for your brothers and sisters, or provided leadership in other ways to extended family members. Whether you are a first-generation student or your family has been in the US for centuries, you may have organized a care-giving network for an ill relative or started a family newsletter that helps people stay in touch. Within every social group, there are leadership opportunities; remember to consider ways you may have exercised leadership in your family as you think about how to demonstrate leadership in your pharmacy school application.

Leadership: pitfalls to avoid

While many students make the mistake of underestimating or understating their leadership experiences and skills, others make the opposite mistake: they overstate their skills in this area or fail to elaborate on why they list an experience as a leadership experience. Some students list "worked as pharmacy technician" as a leadership experience without further comment. In and of itself, working as a pharm tech is not a leadership experience (though if you've been promoted, trained others, or made innovations, it could be described in this way). Some applicants list running in a 5k or a marathon as a leadership experience because they raised some money in association with the event. Running in an American Cancer Society race is a laudable activity, but it isn't in and of itself a leadership experience. If you organize a training group, or hold a community education workshop leading up to the event that focuses on exercise and cancer prevention, this could, however, be seen as a leadership experience. Whether a committee regards your list of leadership activities as "filler" or "substantive" will depend upon both the nature of the activity and how well you convey its leadership aspects. We advise you not to list as leadership an event like "running a 5K" if there are no other leadership elements in the experience, because it will give the impression that you are padding your application. It's likely that you have other experiences that are more impressive in this area—and that you can mention your running accomplishments in another section of your application (the committee will enjoy knowing that you are fitness-minded). Turn to the leadership worksheet at the end of this book to help further define your leadership experiences and goals.

CHAPTER 13
Put Your Best Face Forward: The Interview

Your application to pharmacy school may include interviews on campus at the schools to which you have applied. The interview gives you an opportunity to get a feel for the school and allows the school to get a more three-dimensional sense of who you are—and to evaluate your "communication skills." The interview process can be exciting—and also confusing and stressful. In this chapter, we offer some recommendations for maximizing this opportunity to make a good impression on those who will evaluate you.

Do your homework

One of the most important things you can do to prepare for your pharmacy school interview is to gather as much information as possible about the interview process. You can do this by reviewing the materials the school sends you, by reading about the application process on the school's website, and by asking knowledgeable people about the process. Current and former students are often willing to help, but they may not have the most accurate or up-to-date information on the school's interview process, unless they are part of an interview team or sit on the admissions committee. If you cannot find the answers to your questions in the material the school has already provided you, feel free to make a very polite inquiry of the director of admissions, your advisor in the school (if you currently are a student on that campus and have a pharm school advisor), or someone else you have met who is on the admissions committee—for instance a faculty member who would be aware of current practices. The best resource is no doubt the admissions director or coordinator, but other people can sometimes be helpful as well. Here are some things you want to know:

- Will I be interviewed individually or with other students?
- Who will be conducting the interviews (Faculty? Alumni? Students? Faculty-Alumni teams?)
- Are the interviewers members of the Admissions Committee (or are they volunteers who report their impressions to the Admissions Committee)?

- What is the format or structure of the interview? Upon what will it focus?

- How long will the interview last?

- Are there things I can do to prepare for the interview?

- Is there anything else I should know about the Interview Day—for example, does the school ask for in-house writing samples from applicants coming to the interviews, and will there be opportunities to meet current students during the Interview Day event?

Having the answers to these questions will help put you at ease—you won't be surprised to find yourself in a room with two pharmacists or to be part of a group being interviewed by three faculty members, and you will know how long you can expect to be at the school for your interview. Knowing as much as possible will allow you to envision the interview process ahead of time, and this will make it a more comfortable and exciting experience for you.

Put your research to use

For many interviews, you won't need to do additional homework—it's unlikely that your interviewers are going to ask you about the finer points of calculus. Nonetheless, if you can determine the structure of the interview and its basic content, you can practice ahead of time. For example, if you've been told that two pharmacists will ask you two questions about ethical dilemmas you've experienced, and the interview will take 20 minutes, you can recruit two friends to play the role of pharmacists and ask you about your experiences with ethical issues. If you have determined that you'll be asked about why you want to go to pharmacy school, you can practice conveying your motivations out loud to your friends. Having some practice interviews using what you know from your homework on the process can only build your confidence—which will make your interviews go even better.

Know where you're going and arrive ahead of schedule

Arriving close to the scheduled interview time—or worse yet, late—is a certain way to stress yourself out. Beyond this, it will likely be noted in your application file. Pharmacists value precision, and punctuality is a form of precision. If you live near the place you'll be interviewed but have never been in the building, check it out a few days in advance, so you know where you're going and how to get there ahead of schedule. If you arrive in town the night before the interviews, make walking or driving by a priority for the evening. If you are arriving on the day of the interview, do your best to arrive a couple of hours early. Bring a book, a snack, and your walking shoes so that you can amuse yourself until your interview, but give yourself the comfort of knowing that you don't have to rush and won't be lost when it's time for you to meet with the interviewers or begin the activities of Interview Day.

Dress the part

Unfortunately, some people participating in the process of evaluating you for pharmacy school admission will pay close attention to your attire. Many students are living on limited budgets already strained by the considerable expense of traveling across the country to get to pharmacy school interviews, and may not have much excess in their budgets for an expensive suit. Nonetheless, it is the case that at a pharmacy school interview you will be evaluated not only on your performance but on your appearance, so we would be remiss in not advising you to pay attention to your presentation during the interview experience.

Most applicants adopt a kind of "pharmacy uniform" that essentially consists of a dark suit and light shirt or blouse, with men wearing a tie and women wearing dressy shoes. Pressed khakis and a suit jacket would also work well. It is not necessary to spend a fortune on such an outfit, however. If you feel you must acquire clothes specially for the interview, consider borrowing a suit from a sibling or friend or shopping in a high-quality second-hand clothing store. The most important thing to remember about whatever you wear is that your clothes should be clean and well-ironed, and give the interviewers the impression that you invested some time and energy into dressing "respectfully" for the interview. The times interviewers are likely to make negative comments about an interviewee's appearance are when the applicant looks as though he or she is "dressed for class" or "dressed for a football game" or "dressed for a bar," instead of dressed for professional success. Even though you are applying to a school, the reality is that pharmacy is a profession, and you want to help your interviewers envision you as a young professional in addition to a smart and promising student.

Consistent with "looking professional" as pharmacists define it, women applicants should make sure their tops are not cut low or skirts, if worn, cut high, and men with long hair should make sure their hair is secured away from their faces (though having long hair may still draw comment from interviewers). If you have piercings, it is wise to remove your jewelry, except for standard earrings, and if you have tattoos, it is wise to cover them. If you normally wear your hair a wild shade of blue or green or pink, you may wish to consider returning it to its natural color for interview day.

Be confident... and humble

It is important to communicate that you are happy to be part of the interview process, excited to be considered by this school, eager to take the next step on the road to becoming a pharmacist, and confident that you will work hard and succeed. It is also important, however, to not assume that the interview process is "simply a formality." The interview process has made an impact, both positive and negative, on the outcome of the applications of many people. I recall an applicant who had a 4.0 GPA, excellent PCAT scores, great essays, and research experience—in short, who looked great on paper—who came to the interview in jeans, a leather jacket, and his wallet on a chain, was rude to the person who checked him in, and gave the interviewers the impression that he considered himself a "shoe-in," or certain to be admitted. The person who checked him in reported her experience to the admissions committee, the interviewers recommended against admission, and, despite his great intellect, the applicant was not admitted. On the flip side, a strong positive impression made at the interview has sometimes pushed an applicant who may have been a strong but-not-outstanding applicant on paper into the "we want this student" category. So: take the interview process seriously: don't assume your admission is secure, treat everyone you meet in a respectful, friendly way, and present yourself in as professional a manner as you can muster. Your future may rest in these 20 minutes.

Be aware of cultural differences

In an interview process, you may experience some cross-cultural interactions. If you are interviewing at an institution that is mostly populated by people from your own cultural group, you may feel completely at home, especially if your interviewers are from your cultural and racial background. If you are from a cultural group different from the group to which your interviewers belong, you may experience a cultural disconnection or observe your interviewers being out of their comfort zone in their interactions with you. Although pharmacy schools are working hard to educate their admissions committee members and interviewers about cultural differences, this is still an area in which we all are learning. Because you are an applicant, it is in your best interest to bridge any cultural divide between you and your interviewers.

For example, you may come from a culture in which direct eye contact is seen as disrespectful, but you may be interviewed by people from a cultural background in which direct eye-contact is seen as a sign of respect and good communication. If you show these interviewers respect by not meeting their eyes, they may misinterpret this as shyness, communication difficulty, indirectness, or disrespect. If you are aware that "eye contact" is one of the criteria on which you'll be evaluated, and you come from a culture in which this is not a sign of respect, you may want to practice making eye contact in your rehearsal interviews. This is a skill you will need to learn in order to work well with patients from groups that make a lot of eye contact, so you can consider this part of your cultural preparation.

If you come from a minority cultural group, you likely already have many good skills for navigating cultural differences; nonetheless, this is a time to be especially alert to these. If you come from a majority cultural group and discover yourself being interviewed by people from another cultural background, this is an important opportunity to pay special attention to the cues your interviewers send—and to follow those cues.

Be kind to other applicants

Depending on how the interview process is arranged, you may meet or even spend significant time with other applicants being interviewed on the same day. You may be interviewed with one or more other applicants in a group interview. You only benefit by being kind and helpful to them. They may be your colleague during pharmacy school for the next four years, and they will remember your kindness during your first meeting.

Be prepared to write an in-house essay

While the focus of this essay will likely be something you can address using personal experience, the essay needs to demonstrate thoughtfulness, organization, and attention to detail. Design some practice essay questions for yourself and practice answering them, by hand, with pen and paper, using a standard introductory paragraph/body/concluding paragraph structure. If you haven't had a lot of experience with this in high school and college, seek out training from the writing center on your campus before you go to your pharmacy school interviews.

Check out what other students have said

Use the Student Doctor Network to learn what other students have said about the interview process at the schools that interest you. If you go to www.studentdoctor.net/interview-feedback/, you can choose to read reviews of pharmacy school interviews, organized by school, that tell you the recent questions asked, the applicant's evaluation of the environment, and the applicant's overall assessment of the experience. This isn't a scientific survey, but may give you some sense of the recent interview processes in place at each school.

Remember to go back after your interviews to log your experiences and help others out!

Be excited, be yourself, have fun

Remember that by getting to an interview at a pharmacy school, you have already accomplished your goal of completing a pharmacy school application. The interview is an important opportunity to find out more about your schools of choice, meet people involved in the process, and get a greater sense of what it might mean to be a pharmacy student and, ultimately, a pharmacist. Give yourself credit for what you have achieved, and know that however your applications this year turn out, the experience will be invaluable.

CHAPTER 14

It's Not Over Yet! What To Do While Your App Is Under Review

Believe it or not, putting your pharmacy school applications in the mail or pressing the "send" button to submit your application on-line is not the end of the pharmacy school admissions process! In this chapter, we will give you advice about how to make the most of the waiting period between your application submission and the notification from your schools of choice about your admission status. We'll also make recommendations about what to do if you are admitted—and what to do if you are not admitted this time around.

What to do after you submit your application

If you are still in school, the most important thing for you to do while you are waiting to learn the outcome of your application is to work hard to achieve academic excellence during the current semester. There are three reasons for this:

- You have already established a strong academic track record and know its rewards—maintaining your momentum should be rewarding for the intrinsic value of learning and succeeding as a student.

- Many schools of pharmacy view even positive admissions decisions as "conditional;" if an admitted student's grades drop after she or he has been admitted on paper, the admission may be cancelled, which is heartbreaking! By working hard in the current semester, you make sure this cannot happen to you.

- Because the pharmacy school admissions process is so competitive, it is possible you will not be admitted on your first or even second attempt. If pharmacy is still your goal, you will need to apply in the future. Maintaining or even improving your academic performance while you are awaiting an admissions decision will improve your chances of admission in the coming years.

If you are not currently in school, this is a good period in which to make plans for the following year: Plan A should center on how your life will change if you are admitted to pharmacy school; Plan B should center on how you will move forward if you are not admitted this year. If you are a working adult student, a student with a family, or a student who has been out of school for several years, starting pharmacy school will mean many changes for you, socially, financially, and in terms of your schedule. Now is a good time to consider what you will need to do to have a balanced life as you make the transition.

What to do if you are admitted to pharmacy school

First, of course, accept our congratulations! You have achieved something extraordinary through your hard work—and it has earned you the opportunity to do even more hard work in the coming years! We hope you take an evening to celebrate now, and plan a longer celebration in the future, when you know your admission is secure.

If you are a current student: you must continue to work hard to finish up the current semester in great standing. There will be time to relax after the end of the semester, but during this last semester before pharmacy school, it is crucial that you work hard to maintain your GPA. We have known people who have been admitted, only to have their admissions cancelled because they encountered academic difficulty (and this could mean only earning a B– in a class!) in the last semester before they would have enrolled. This meant that they had to apply to pharmacy school again in the coming years. In some instances, they were able to recover and gain admission; unfortunately, in others, the competition the following year was tougher, or their academic troubles worried the committee enough that they were not admitted when they applied again. Don't let this happen to you!

If you are fortunate enough to be admitted to more than one Pharm.D. program, you will need to make decisions by the announced deadline about which school you will attend and which schools you will decide against. In this situation, remember that someone else, just as eager to be a pharmacist as you, is on a waiting list and will only be able to go to pharmacy school after you have relinquished your seat. If you are deciding against a school, it is courteous, kind, and professional to inform that school as early as possible. If you need more information from a school about tuition, housing, scholarships, loans, or other issues, contact the appropriate person at the school to ask these questions. In the back of this chapter, we have included a list of issues to consider when deciding between two or more schools; feel free to use this when you are deliberating and asking questions.

Your school/s will inform you about your acceptance deadline. Again, it is wise to confirm with the school before the deadline. Failure to do so could cost you your place in the incoming class—or could get you off to a bumpy start with your advisor or the admissions chair, which could have consequences for you down the road.

If your plans have changed or something has come up in your life that makes it impossible or difficult for you to come to pharmacy school for the year you have been admitted, you don't necessarily have to begin anew. Some schools will allow you to defer your admission for a year for a good reason. Before you simply decline because you're facing tough circumstances or need to prolong your undergraduate coursework to finish a second degree, it may be worth asking if you can defer for a year.

What to do if you are on the "Wait List" or "Alternate List"

Some schools—those that admit a whole cohort at once, instead of on a rolling basis—will set aside a group of applicants for a "wait list." If your application is on the wait list, it means that the school may still admit you for the following year, if spaces in the in-coming class open up. That might happen early in the admissions process, when a student who has been admitted elsewhere decides to decline admission to your school of choice; it may happen closer to the beginning of fall semester, when a student in the admitted class realizes that she or he is going to be unable to attend after all. If you are on the "wait list," ask the admissions director your rank on the list and how many from the list were admitted last year, but be prepared that the admissions director may decline to tell you your exact ranking. This may give you some sense of the probability of your being admitted to this school this year. If you are not admitted ultimately, and have not accepted admission somewhere else, follow the steps outlined below for declined applications. Know, however, that having your name on the wait list is a sign that you are definitely on the right track. If you are admitted from the wait list, trust that your qualifications are just as strong as those in the rest of your cohort, and that there is no difference between students admitted from the wait list and students admitted earlier.

What to do if your application is declined

Unfortunately, there are many more applications to most pharmacy programs than there are seats for students in those programs. This means that every year, pharmacy schools turn away more applicants than they can accept. And while it is true that some applicants simply aren't yet well prepared to succeed in pharmacy school, it is also true that the vast majority of applicants probably have the potential to succeed. While my colleagues and I always felt good about the applicants we could admit, we also often felt very sad and frustrated about those we had to turn away because we simply didn't have room in the school for more students. Often, I heard my colleagues express during our deliberations their hope that a student would apply again in the coming year or years, because they could see the achievements and potential so common among those we had to turn away.

If your application was not accepted on your first attempt, and pharmacy is still your goal, don't give up.

If your application has been declined, you will very likely be disappointed. This is normal. How you handle your disappointment will make a difference in your future success, so here is what we are going to recommend you do:

- Give yourself a few days to process the outcome of your application and to work through your feelings in a healthy way.

- Continue to apply yourself diligently to your current classes if you are now a student; if you are going to apply again, the committee will be looking at this semester's grades, and they will be important.

- When you feel you can do this in a productive way, contact the admissions official at the school that has declined your application and make a phone appointment or in-person appointment with him or her.

- During your appointment, have the goals of 1) finding out what you can do to improve your application the next time you submit it and 2) impressing the admissions director with how gracefully and maturely you handle this disappointment.

- Take good notes during your appointment; listen carefully and ask good questions; assume that the person with whom you are meeting is doing his or her best to give you helpful information.

If, after you meet with an advisor or admissions director who can give you specific information about how to improve your pharmacy application, you decide you would like to apply again, it is imperative that you take the advice you've received very seriously. Follow through on any suggestion the admissions director or advisor has made. There are two reasons to do this. First, the person has likely given you very good advice. Second, a note will be added to your application file about this meeting, and it will tell the next committee that reviews your file next year what you were encouraged to do. When a second-time applicant's materials appear before the committee, the committee will want to see both the improvements you have made and that you have taken the school's recommendations seriously. If you have done what the school directed successfully, the committee has a harder time declining your application a second time.

If you cannot at present accomplish what the school is recommending as an improvement, hold off on any subsequent applications until you can. For example, if the school representative says the committee would like to see you improve your grades in upper-level science classes, it will not work in your favor if you re-take the science classes but earn grades only marginally better than those you've earned before. If you are working many hours or have intense family obligations that prevent you from earning A's in the classes the committee wants you to take or re-take, it is best to wait until the conditions in your life allow you to do exactly what the committee has suggested or requested.

You may also decide after meeting with a representative from the school that it's time for you to explore your alternative career plans. Having done your research earlier, you know that there are many possible career paths for you, given your interests in science, health, and health care. A skilled pharmacy school advisor, an undergraduate advisor, a knowledgeable faculty member, a staff member in the career counseling office at your school, or a personal academic or career coach may also help you assess your strengths and interests and further explore allied health professions that may be good choices for you if you decide that pharmacy school is not for you.

CHAPTER 15
Notes From a Happy Young Pharmacist

Kajua Lor, Pharm.D.

Throughout my childhood and teenage years, I aspired to become a teacher, architect and interior designer. Eventually, I was fortunate to be introduced to the pharmacy profession through my uncle, who was a pharmacy technician at an independent pharmacy. As a first-generation Hmong-American student, I became interested in the work that my uncle recommended I consider. During high school, I was invited to a social "pharmacy" dinner. The pharmacist who was there asked me, "What are your strengths?" I told him that I always had excelled at science and math; he replied that pharmacy would be a great profession for me. After that dinner, I started to do more research about pharmacy. I learned about the changing face of the pharmacy profession from a dispensing field to one in which pharmacists are sitting down with patients to talk about their medicines. So, if I entered the profession of pharmacy, not only would I be able to use my strengths in science and math, but I would also be able to educate patients about their medicines. I decided that I would go on the path to becoming a pharmacist.

During high school, I took many Advanced Placement and college courses, including psychology, calculus, chemistry and Spanish. These courses helped me when I got to the University of Wisconsin because I arrived at college with credits already on my transcript. In high school, as a volunteer for the Red Cross, I was involved in several community events raising money for good causes, being involved in food pantries, and walking to raise funds for leukemia research. During my undergraduate years, I continued to be involved in service work by travelling to Baltimore, Maryland for Habitat for Humanity. I was fortunate to obtain a position as the UW Pre-School of Pharmacy Club president, which cemented my interest in the profession, helped me develop leadership skills, and let me meet other pre-pharmacy students, as well as faculty members and advisors.

In my pharmacy school application, I stated that my main goal was to bridge the gap between modern Western and traditional Hmong medicine, which focuses on the use of "green medicine" or "healing plants" to improve people's health. In my first years of college, I started to explore my identity as a Hmong-American. I became interested in Hmong culture, health beliefs, and herbal medicine when

I worked as an undergraduate research assistant on a Hmong Research Project in the Linguistics Department. I interviewed four and five year old Hmong children on speech and linguistics. I continued to stay involved in the Hmong community by serving as the United Refugee Services of Wisconsin pageant coordinator. Taking a summer-long UW Southeast Asian American Studies Institute(SEASSI) course on Hmong history and culture deepened my interest in the Hmong culture, health beliefs and herbal medicine.

When I applied to pharmacy school, I didn't know how I would bridge the gap between Green Medicine and amber-colored pill bottles, but I knew that going to pharmacy school would give me the scientific knowledge, research skills, and clinical experience that would point me in the right direction. During pharmacy school, in addition to the traditional Western curriculum, I found ways to explore traditional healing using the tools of Western research and the clinical experiences provided by the UW School of Pharmacy. For example, the summer after my second year in pharmacy school, I arranged an independent study that let me develop a video documentary on herbal medicine with my great grandmother, who was a shaman and herbal healer. In my third year, my colleague Kashea Lovaj and I transcribed and translated the video. With these results, we published an article in the Journal of the Pharmacy Society of Wisconsin. I shared my results at the state Pharmacy Society of Wisconsin Educational Conference and at the 2009 national American Pharmacist Association (APhA) Annual Meeting in San Antonio, TX. At the 2009 PSW educational conference, I delivered a presentation on "Cultural Perspective: Hmong and Pharmacy" and shared the Hmong culture and health beliefs with pharmacists and pharmacy students from across the state of Wisconsin. With all these experiences, I was able to work further towards my goal of bridging the gap between Hmong and Western medicine.

I learned in pharmacy school that I enjoyed patient care and being able to interact with doctors and nurses. I was introduced to Medication Therapy Management (MTM) services during one of my internships. I currently hold a pharmaceutical care resident position at the University of Minnesota–College of Pharmacy Ambulatory Care Residency Program and am on my way to becoming a Medication Therapy Management (MTM) Pharmacist working at an international clinic in the Twin Cities area. There, I will be able to serve Hmong and Spanish-speaking patients, and put to good use my cross-cultural health care and clinical skills. Six years ago, this was my dream. Now, I am able to provide culturally competent pharmacy care to Hmong and Spanish-speaking patients and pursue my passion of bridging the gap between western and Hmong medicine.

There are endless possibilities for what you can do with your Pharm.D. career. The process of getting into pharmacy school is tough. You will need strong grades, a good interview, and experience in several areas of life significant to the profession of pharmacy. Once you're in the door, pharmacy school itself will be very demanding, but finishing pharmacy school will be one of the most rewarding accomplishments you will achieve. This book begins with an essay on why pharmacists are happy with their career choices. I hope you can tell from my experiences why I am both proud and happy to be a member of the profession of pharmacy, and why I wanted to help write this book; if pharmacy is your chosen profession, I hope our advice and experience can help you on the path toward your goal of getting into pharmacy school. A rewarding and happy career awaits!

CHAPTER 16
Worksheets

Worksheet 1: Assessing Careers in the Health Professions

There are many interesting and high-paying careers in the health professions. The foundation you are creating in preparation for pharmacy school is probably also a good foundation for many other careers. Explore them! Use this worksheet to list the positives and negatives (if any) of each of the following areas in health care. Do some research on each profession and determine the following for each one:

PAY	HOURS
INTELLECTUAL STIMULATION	DEMAND FOR WORKERS IN THIS CAREER
CAREER FLEXIBILITY	WORKER SATISFACTION
FAMILY-FRIENDLINESS	STRESS LEVEL
DIVERSITY	YEARS OF TRAINING REQUIRED
WORK ENVIRONMENT	PERSONAL INTERACTION LEVEL
ABILITY TO HELP PEOPLE	ABILITY TO AFFECT HEALTH CARE SYSTEMS
VARIETY OF POSSIBLE JOBS	

OTHER FACTORS IMPORTANT TO YOU: _____

Using the variables above, record what you see as the positives and negatives of each profession on the worksheet below. Use your findings to think more about your interest in pharmacy and about other careers that are appealing to you within the health professions.

Profession	Positives	Negatives
Nursing		
Public Health		
Physicians Assistant		
Pharmaceutical Research		

Profession	Positives	Negatives
Medical Social Work		
Medicine		
Veterinary Medicine		
Physical Therapy		
Occupational Therapy		
Respiratory Therapy		
Radiation Technology		
Ultrasound Technology		
Dentistry		
Phlebotomy		
Healthcare/ Hospital Administration		
Health Care Information Systems Design And Management (Computer/Information Technology)		
Chiropractic		
Opthamology		

Worksheet 2: Pharmacy

Research these factors as they relate to the profession of pharmacy. Jot some details after each item, and then mark each item with a (+) or (-) sign to indicate whether you like what you have discovered about this variable in careers in pharmacy.

(+) or (-) ?

PAY

HOURS

INTELLECTUAL STIMULATION

DEMAND FOR WORKERS IN THIS CAREER

CAREER FLEXIBILITY

WORKER SATISFACTION

FAMILY-FRIENDLINESS

STRESS LEVEL

DIVERSITY

YEARS OF TRAINING REQUIRED

WORK ENVIRONMENT

PERSONAL INTERACTION LEVEL

ABILITY TO HELP PEOPLE

ABILITY TO AFFECT HEALTH CARE SYSTEMS

VARIETY OF POSSIBLE JOBS

OTHER FACTORS IMPORTANT TO YOU:

Worksheet 3: What Do Pharmacy Schools Want?

Use this chart to determine what is required of applicants at three schools of pharmacy that interest you, then use this information to make a plan for fulfilling their requirements.

School	GPA	PCAT	Letters	Diversity	Leadership	Healthcare	Application Due Date
1)							
2)							
3)							

COURSES REQUIRED

School	Science	Math	Social science	Humanities
1)				
2)				
3)				

Worksheet 4: Health Care Experience Tracker

Formal positions I have held in health care settings:

Volunteer jobs I have held in health care:

Training I have had related to health care (CPR, etc):

Shadowing experiences I have had in health care settings:

Interviews I have conducted with health care practitioners:

Patient populations with which I'm familiar (people with disabilities, elders, people from a particular ethnic group):

Alternative/traditional approaches to medicine and health care I know about:

Classes I've taken and class projects I have done related to health care:

Personal and family experiences I have had related to health care:

Worksheet 5: Assessing and Improving Cultural Competence

The first thing to do in assessing your cultural competence is to make sure you know yourself. Here are some qualities for you to notice about yourself:

Age:

Sex:

Gender:

Race/s:

Ethnicities:

Languages:

Class background:

Parents' educational background:

Parents' professions:

Religion/spirituality:

Family size:

Extended family size:

How many cultural groups are represented in your extended family?

How many cultural groups are represented in the neighborhood in which you grew up?

With which group do you identify most closely (circle one):
my race   my religion   my class   my ethnicity   my language group
my nationality   my sports teams   my family   my state my clan
my tribe my neighborhood   my classmates   my profession

Ways in which I am sometimes in the minority:
by race   by class   by religion   by sexual identity   by nationality
by disability or handicap   by language   by sex/gender

SECTION 2: Cross-cultural strengths: Which of the following is true of you?

__ I have friends and family members from a variety of cultural groups

__ I speak more than one language

__ I have traveled beyond my hometown/state/region/country

__ I have worked/studied with people whose cultural habits and values are different from my own

__ I have read about the history of people from cultural groups different from my own

__ I have attended a gay pride march, a Christian wedding, a Buddhist meditation circle, a Hmong cultural festival, a Southern Baptist worship service, a fundamentalist prayer breakfast, a formal dance, a community health clinic, and other similar events to find out about what people different from me care about

__ When I can, I attend community and campus programming on diversity issues

__ I have designed class projects for myself that allow me to interview health care providers about the cultural issues that come up in their work

SECTION THREE: A plan to expand
Below, identify three classes you could take that would improve your cultural competence:

1.

2.

3.

Below, identify three cultural groups that especially interest you:

1.

2.

3.

Below, identify three resources you could use to find out more about the health care issues and experiences of the groups you have just named:

1.

2.

3.

Worksheet 6: 50 Ways to Enhance Your Cultural Competence

The social world is a fascinating place, full of immense opportunities for life-long learning. Health care professionals increasingly seek opportunities to deepen their awareness of cultural and social diversity in their commitment to providing the best possible care to as many people as possible. No single event, course, or experience makes us culturally sophisticated or sensitive; embracing many opportunities over the course of our lifetimes allows us to more deeply understand the remarkable connections and the rich differences among people. Here, we offer a short, general list of *some* experiences *some* people have found exciting, interesting, and valuable in their efforts to become more culturally competent. We hope they inspire you! Circle 10 that interest you!

1. Learn a foreign language
2. Use your foreign language in community service
3. Study abroad
4. Take a course in anthropological fieldwork
5. Serve as a host, tutor, or goodwill ambassador to people from another country
6. Tutor minority kids
7. Volunteer at a minority health fair
8. Take courses in Black History, Chicano Studies, Women's Studies, Asian-American Studies, Sociology, and Anthropology
9. Read history and sociology texts written by women and people of color
10. Make cross-cultural friendship
11. Organize a multicultural event
12. Diversify an organization to which you belong
13. Undertake a research project on a cultural group different from your own
14. Study white privilege
15. Produce a cultural portfolio documenting your own family's cultural history
16. Travel
17. Put yourself in situations that allow you to be in the minority
18. Familiarize yourself with the musical traditions of your cultural group and those of others
19. Learn the history of several forms of dance—and how to do them
20. Study the world's religions
21. Take a course on global politics or global environmental studies.
22. Volunteer at a minority health clinic or an HIV education program
23. Volunteer at an LGBT community Center
24. Join a LGBT&Allies group—or form a Gay-Straight Alliance at your high school

25. Volunteer in a community health clinic or VA hospital

26. Join an organization working to end racism

27. Help organize Black, Latino, Asian, Native American, or Women's History Month activities at your school

28. Volunteer with refugees

29. Participate in an organization that provides social services to minority community

30. Organize a film series around religious, cultural, ethnic, or racial diversity

31. Watch the Black history documentary series *Eyes on the Prize*

32. Study ethnobotany

33. Learn the history of and how to cook the food of another cultural group (after you've learned to cook the food of your own community!)

34. Read, read, read!

35. Become the pen-pal of someone in another country

36. Volunteer at an ethic community festival, celebration, or pow-wow

37. Become involved in a political initiative related to minority, women's, or LGBT interests

38. Form or participate in a theatre-of-the-oppressed or diversity-oriented theatre project

39. Organize or participate in a disability awareness program

40. Educate yourself and then your peers about hate speech

41. Initiate LGBT safe-space programming in your school or workplace

42. Organize, attend, or participate in a krystal nacht or holocaust remembrance event

43. Attend religious services, lectures, or celebrations of spiritual traditions different from your own

44. Learn sign language

45. Make your school, workplace, or residence hall a violence & harassment free zone

46. Volunteer at a women's shelter, homeless shelter, or food bank

47. Learn the games of other cultures

48. Read the alternative press; discover free speech radio news

49. Learn karate, aikido, yoga, meditation, shiatsu, t'ai chi, qi gong, or another form of Eastern energy work

50. Study conflict resolution; teach others; bring strategies for ethnic harmony to the places you live and work

Worksheet 7: My Leadership Experiences and Skills

Use the following tables to track your leadership experiences:

Formal Leadership

Organization	Role/Position	Major Accomplishments/Activities	Years
1.			
2.			
3.			
4.			
5.			

EX: School Newspaper, Asst Editor, Recruited and trained new writers, 2009–2011

Informal Leadership

Issue or Need: Example: Students in my chem. class were failing

How I got involved: Example: Organized three study circles with support of my professor; arranged rooms and times; arranged TA to visit with each group once a week; all participants passed the class!

Issue or Need:

How I got involved:

Issue or Need:

How I got involved:

Issue or Need:

How I got involved:

Worksheet 8: Questions to Ask if You Are Deciding Between Two Schools

	School 1	School 2
Cost/year		
Financial aid/support		
Is this school accredited?		
Where is each of these schools ranked among schools in the nation?		
Quality of life for people like me (i.e. housing, social networks, student organizations, health care on campus)?		
How many other people from my group (students of color, people from other countries, people from my ethnic group, women, people with disabilities) go to this school?		
How many of the students who start this program finish? What is the graduation rate? What is known about the students who don't finish?		
What percentage of the graduates of this school pass their pharmacy licensing exams on the first try?		
Does this school offer some training in areas of specialization that interest me?		
Will my significant other be able to find work in this town?		
Will my kids and significant others feel welcome in this school/ community?		
Do I have the general impression that people in this school are happy?		

	School 1	School 2
Is there a special requirement for the pharmacy state licensing exam? (i.e., consultation exam, compounding exam) ?		
How many pharmacy schools are in this state?		
What organizations could you get involved with at the school? Do they interest you?		
Educational resources (labs, libraries, study areas)		

References and Resources

American Association of Colleges of Pharmacy website
www.aacp.org

Close the Gaps Cultural Consulting website
www.closethegapsculturalconsulting.com

Figg, William Douglas & Chau, Cindy H. 2009. *Get Into Pharmacy School: RX for Success!* New York: Kaplan Publishing

Halbur, Kimberly Vess & Halbur, Duane A. 2008. *Essentials of Cultural Competence in Pharmacy Practice.* Washington, D.C.: American Pharmacists Association

Nemko, Marty. 2008. "Best Careers 2009: Pharmacist." U.S. News & World Report: Dec. 11, 2008. www.usnews.com/money/careers/articles/2008/12/11/best-careers-2009-pharmacist.html

Pharmacy College Admissions Test
www.pcatweb.info

Pharmacy Insider
www.rxinsider.com/schools_of_pharmacy.htm

Student Doctor Network
www.student-doctor.net/interview-feedback/

SQ3R Study Strategy website
www.studygs.net/texred2.htm

US Bureau of Labor Statistics Occupational Outlook Handbook website
www.bls.gov/k12/index.htm